Otmane CHEKROUN

Treatment of respiratory distress

Otmane CHEKROUN

Treatment of respiratory distress

ScienciaScripts

Contents

Dedication

I dedicate this work to :
My wife and children Nour El Houda, Allaa Sarah, Farah and Imad
Abdelrahmane.
My whole family

Why this book

This book is intended for general practitioners, emergency physicians, medical interns and medical students to complement their knowledge of our respiratory system, from its formation during the embryonic phase right up to birth, and to provide them with knowledge of the functioning and pathophysiology of this system and the various causes of respiratory distress, thereby facilitating pre-hospital and hospital management of patients suffering from respiratory insufficiency.

Our respiratory system is so exposed to different types of aggression (viral, bacterial, traumatic, ...) that any pathology of this system can compromise the transport and use of oxygen by the cell, thereby endangering our organism.

Enjoy your reading.

Otmane CHEKROUN

Chapter 1
Introduction

Respiratory distress is one of the most frequent causes of calls to the emergency medical service. Elie presents with an acute respiratory condition that may be life-threatening. Among the most common causes: bronchial asthma, COPD decompensation, strange bodies in children, OAP, pneumothorax, chest trauma, requiring treatment adapted to the cause and medical transport by the EMS.

Acute respiratory failure is a syndrome defined by an acute alteration in hematosis related to the failure of one or more components of the respiratory system (airways, pulmonary parenchyma, pleura, vessels, respiratory muscles and respiratory control). A distinction is made between :

• acute hypoxemic respiratory failure or type I respiratory failure defined by a partial pressure of oxygen in the arterial blood (PaO2) < 60 mm Hg;

• Acute hypercapnic or type II respiratory failure, characterised by a partial pressure of carbon dioxide in the arterial blood (PaO2) > 45 mm Hg, combined with a fall in blood pH reflecting respiratory acidosis.

This definition is an operational definition (usable in clinical practice), because it is based on the measurement of arterial blood gases, but it is restrictive in that it excludes tissue hypoxia without hypoxemia (which can only be detected in practice indirectly by measuring arterial lactate) linked to an alteration in the transport of oxygen (anaemia, carbon monoxide poisoning, shock states, etc.) or to an alteration in cellular respiration (cyanide poisoning, severe sepsis, etc.)..) or altered cellular respiration (cyanide poisoning, severe sepsis....). Acute respiratory failure can also be defined more broadly as the acute onset of tissue hypoxia.

In addition, the term "hypercapnic acute respiratory failure" is inappropriate in the absence of hypoxemia and should be more strictly replaced by the term "acute ventilatory failure".

Frequent confusion between the notion of "respiratory distress" and "adult acute respiratory distress syndrome" or ARDS.

Respiratory distress" is a group of signs indicating the seriousness of a respiratory condition.

ARDS is a syndrome resulting from a lesional collapse of the lung, of which there are many causes;

Chapter 2
Embryology

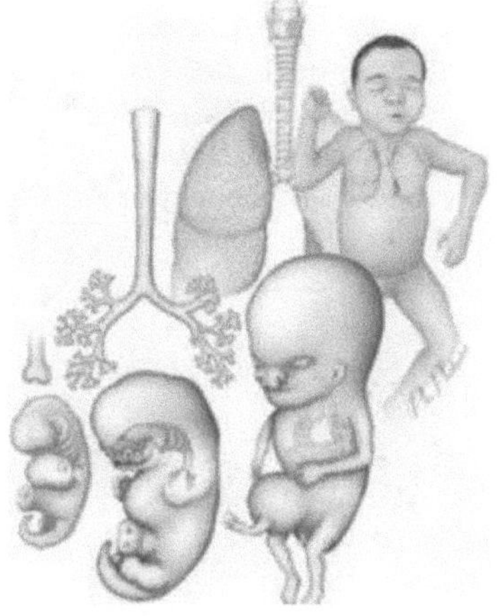

2.1   Airway formation

2.1.1 The respiratory diverticulum

The respiratory diverticulum appears at 4 weeks in the form of a groove on the ventral surface of the caudal part of the pharyngeal intestine. This groove, open at the back, separates from the primitive intestine which gave birth to it, due to the proliferation of two zones of mesenchyme which insert themselves between the two structures and progress in a caudal direction. The embryo then forms a straight tube, blind at the caudal end, which communicates with the cavity of the pharyngeal intestine at the cephalic end. This communication orifice becomes the laryngeal orifice, separated from the base of the tongue by the epiglottis.

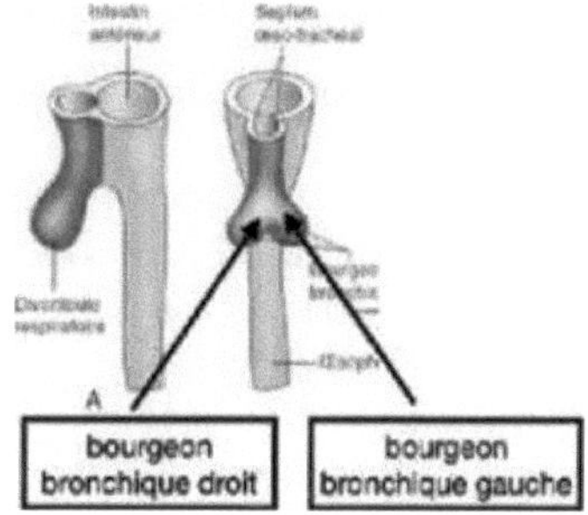

Figure 2.2

2.1.2 Bronchial buds

As soon as it is individualised, the respiratory diverticulum divides at its caudal end into two buds, the right and left bronchial buds, which give rise to the stem branches, while the straight segment gives rise to the trachea.

During the 5th week, the bronchial buds divide in turn, but asymmetrically: on the left, the bronchial bud divides into two secondary bronchial buds corresponding to the future left lobar branches, whereas on the right, the bronchial bud gives rise to three buds corresponding to the future right lobar branches.

From then on, the lobar buds will undergo successive division into two branches (dichotomous mode) which will give rise, between the 5th and 17th weeks, to bronchial elements whose calibre decreases with each division. This mechanism results in the formation of all the airways from the lobar branches to the bronchioles (17th order divisions), although there are frequent individual variations. The last divisions may occur after birth.

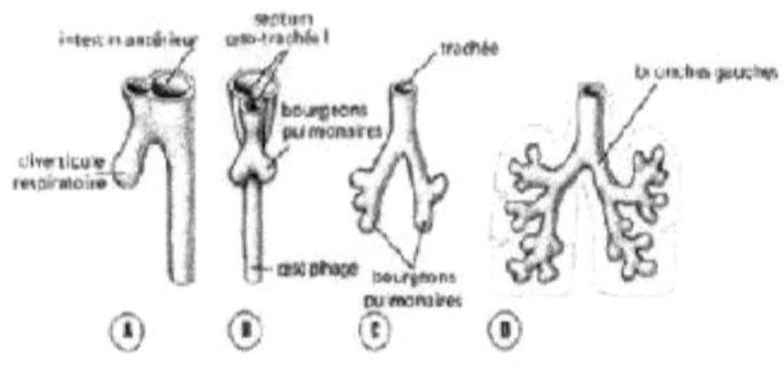

FIGURE 2.3

2.1.3 Airway walls

The walls of the airways result from the differentiation of the mesenchyme in contact with the end of the buds as a result of a reciprocal endoderm/mesenchyme induction mechanism. This differentiation gives rise to the components of the walls: connective, muscular and cartilaginous tissues, which take on different appearances depending on the calibre of the bronchus.

2.2 Formation of the lung parenchyma

The lung parenchyma gradually builds up around the airways, leading to the description of four successive overlapping periods depending on the stage of development and histological appearance.

2.2.1 The pseudo-glandular period

The pseudo-glandular period corresponds to the formation of the airways up to the bronchioles (from the 5th to the 17th week). These are lined by cubic epithelium, with rare alveoli in the so-called respiratory bronchioles.

2.2.2 The root canal period

The ductal period corresponds to the appearance of the alveolar ducts (from the 17th to the 25th week): the numerous alveoli circumscribe the duct, the lumen of which is bordered by flattened epithelium at the level of the thin inter-alveolar partitions.

2.2.3 The terminal bag period

The "terminal sac" period corresponds to the formation of the first alveolar sacs made up of juxtaposed alveoli (the bronchial border is no longer present). This period begins around the 24th week, during which the alveolar cells (type II pneumocytes) begin to secrete surfactant. The number of alveoli and the maturation of the secreted product allow a premature baby to survive from the 26th week.

2.2.4 The alveolar period

The alveolar period corresponds to the end of pregnancy and continues beyond birth. It is characterised by the formation of the definitive alveolar sacs and the progressive increase in lung volume.

The very small spaces remaining between the alveoli are occupied by the remains of the mesenchyme which will give a fine connective tissue, the interstitium, where the blood vessels run.

2.3   Formation of blood vessels

2.3.1 The vessels before the second month

Before the second month: At the time of Γ individualisation of the respiratory diverticulum, its vascularisation depends on that of the primitive anterior intestine from which it derives. There is an afferent plexus coming from the ventral branches of the dorsal aortas and an efferent network drained by the branches of the anterior cardinal veins. These networks branch into the mesenchyme tracts as the airways branch and the parenchyma is organised.

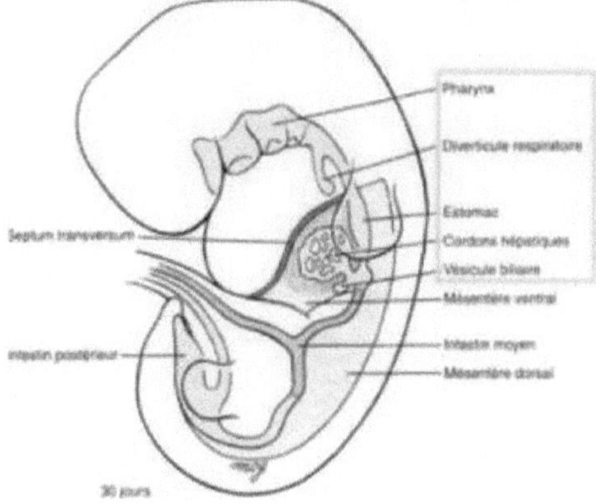

FIGURE 2.4

2.3.2 During the second month

During the second month: the afferent and efferent vessels will change:

1.   Segmentation of the conotruncus results in the formation of the pulmonary artery trunk, which communicates with the proximal part of the sixth left aortic arch. This new afferent pathway terminates at the initial plexus of the respiratory diverticulum, where it becomes the dominant source constituting the pulmonary artery pathway. The afferent branches from the dorsal aortas regress, except for the most cranial, which become the bronchial arteries.

2.   The dorsal wall of the atrium gives rise to four evaginations (two on the right and two on the left) which connect with the efferent network of the pulmonary artery. These evaginations correspond to the pulmonary veins which preferentially drain the efferent circulation towards the left atrium. Some of the primitive veins of the saphenous vein persist and become the bronchial veins which drain into the superior vena cava. From this point onwards, the lower respiratory tract is the site of a dual circulation, one passing through the pulmonary vessels and the other through the bronchial vessels. During the rest of the pregnancy, this circulation remains solely nourishing, with gas exchange taking place at the level of the placenta.

2.3.3 At birth

At birth: The newborn's first cries and respiratory movements cause the alveoli to swell and expand, bringing the pneumocytes lining their lumen into contact with the walls of the capillaries in the interstitium and allowing respiratory exchanges to take place. The pulmonary circulation becomes functional and drains oxygenated blood towards the heart, while the bronchial circulation has only a nourishing role.

Chapter 3
Anatomy of the respiratory system

3.1 Introduction

The role of the lungs is to ensure the exchange of carbon dioxide and oxygen between ambient Fair and the human body. On inspiration, Fair arrives via the trachea and is distributed into the bronchi, then the bronchioles, and finally the alveoli. The oxygen contained in Fair passes through the walls of the alveoli into the blood. The blood then distributes the oxygen to all the body's cells. At the same time, in the opposite direction, the carbon dioxide released by the body's cells passes through the alveoli, then the bronchioles and finally the bronchi. It escapes through the trachea and then through the nose and mouth. This is called exhalation.

3.2 Airways

The airway is the set of ducts through which Fair travels to the lungs. Classically, a distinction is made between the upper airways above the larynx and the lower airways below. Elies include :

- the nasal cavity
- the pharynx, which comprises 3 zones:
— the nasopharynx,
— Foropharynx,
— Fhypopharynx,
- mouth,
- the larynx
- The ear is connected to the nasopharynx by the Eustachian tube.

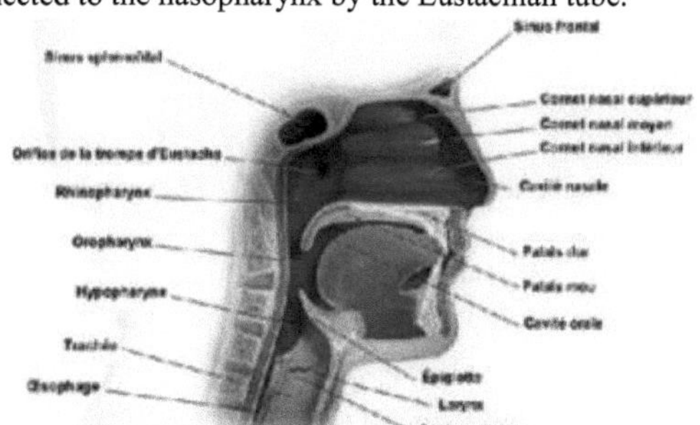

FIGURE 3.1 - The upper airways

The lower airways consist of the trachea, bronchi, bronchioles and pulmonary alveoli (tracheobronchial tree).

The trachea is a tube held aloft by twenty or so rings of cartilage and leads Fair from the larynx to the bronchi.

The bronchi are the ducts that carry Fair from the trachea to each lung. When the muscle surrounding the bronchi contracts, it can alter the diameter of the bronchi, known as bronchoconstriction.

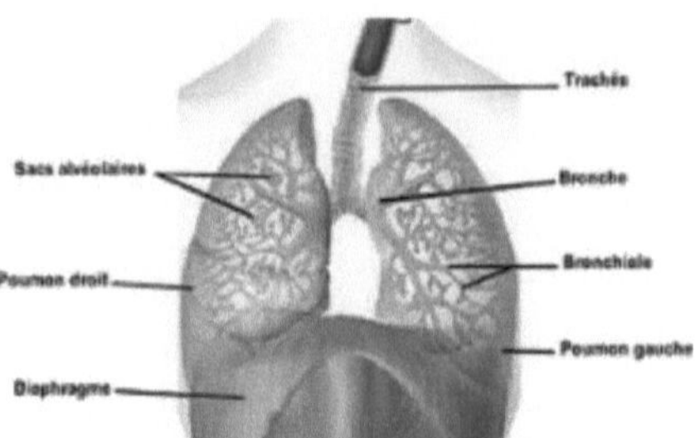

FIGURE 3.2 - The lower airways

The terminal branching of the bronchi is called a bronchiole. The bronchioles have no cartilage, are thin like hairs and end in tiny air-filled sacs: the pulmonary alveoli. A pulmonary alveolus is a small, thin-walled air-filled sac located at the lextremite of the bronchioles, where respiratory gas exchange takes place.

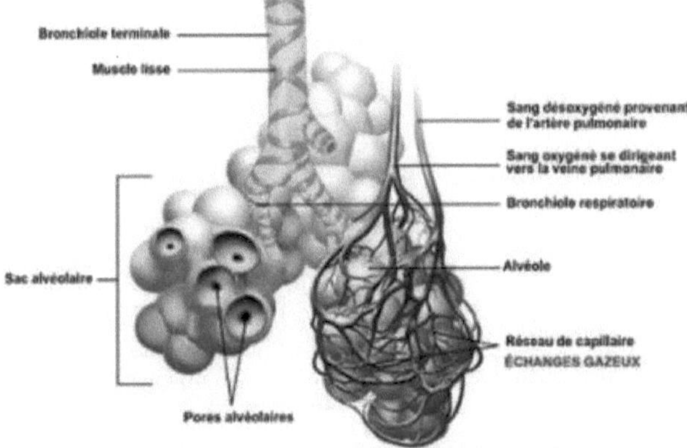

FIGURE 3.3 - The lower airways

The lungs are spongy, voluminous and conical organs. They are made up of bronchioles, alveoli and pulmonary capillaries.

The pleura is made up of two layers, one in contact with the inside wall of the chest and the other in contact with the lungs. Between the two layers of the pleura there is a tiny amount of fluid (pleural fluid) which allows the two layers to slide over each other.

3.3 Radioanatomy of the thorax

The aim of thoracic radioanatomy is to visualise the main anatomical elements that make up the respiratory system and mediastinum.

The paraclinical examination consists of :

1) standard chest X-rays

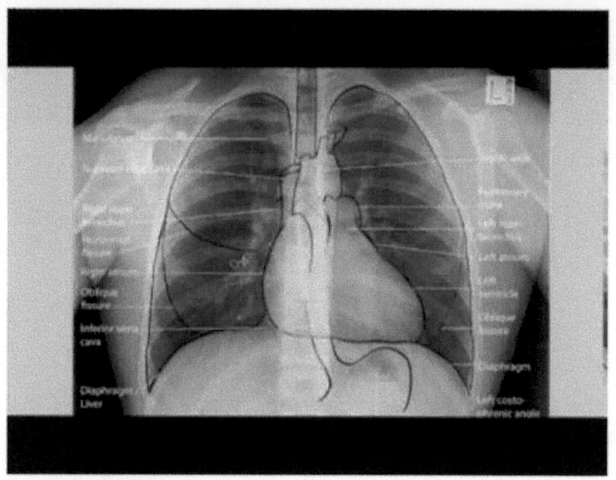

FIGURE 3.4 - Standard chest X-ray

2) Chest scan with or without injections

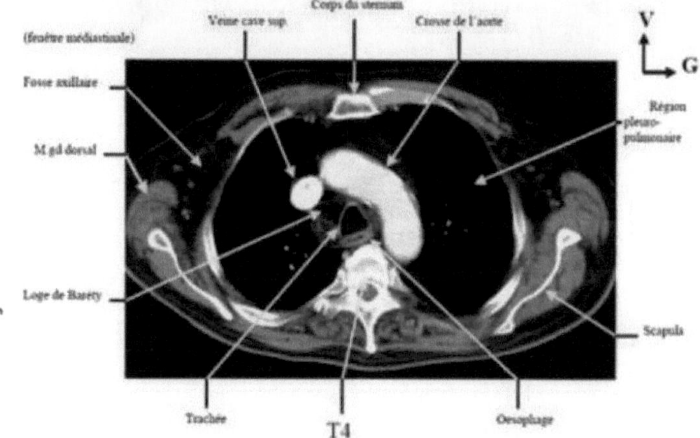

FIGURE 3.5 - Chest CT scan

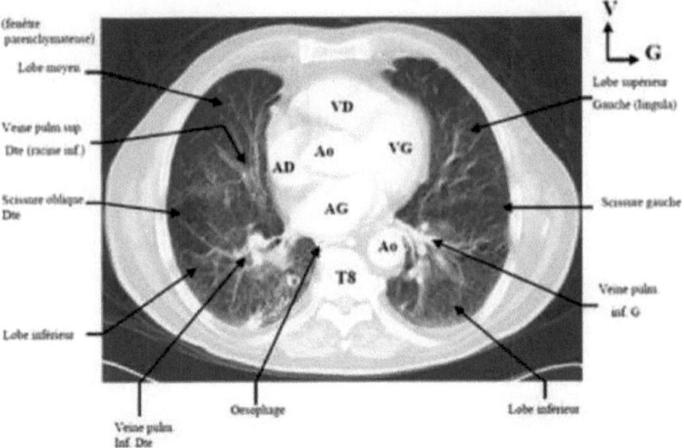

FIGURE 3.6 - Chest CT scan

3) magnetic resonance imaging.

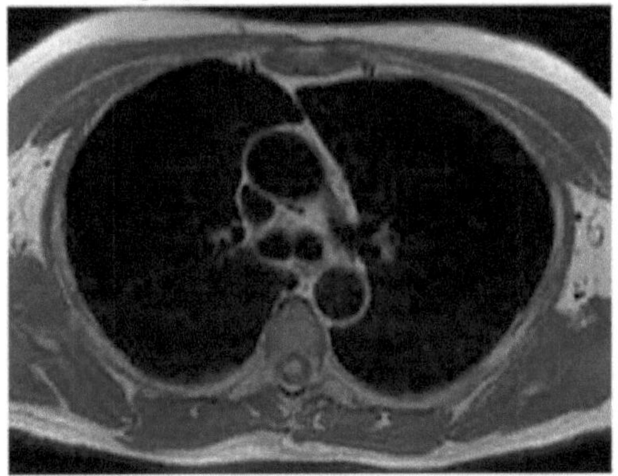

FIGURE 3.7 - Thoracic MRI and MRI angiography

Chapter 4
Physiology of the respiratory system

4.1 Introduction

Blood transports nutrients, hormones, waste products, heat and respiratory gases o dioxygen (O2) and carbon dioxide (CO_2). It is an intermediary transport medium between the external environment and the body's cells.

Gas exchange is essential for the renewal of blood gases.

•   Atmospheric $ΓO2$ is taken up by the blood in the pulmonary alveoli and transported to the cells (organs).

• $CO2$ is taken up by the blood in the cells (organs) and transported to the pulmonary alveoli.

The transport of O_2 and $CO2$ depends on 4 distinct processes:

•   pulmonary ventilation (movement of gases in and out of the lungs)

•   alveolar-capillary diffusion

•   blood transport of O_2 and $CO2$

•   the passage of gases from the capillaries to the tissues (cellular respiration)

Hematosis is the enrichment of blood in O2 and its depletion in CO_2 , in the lungs.

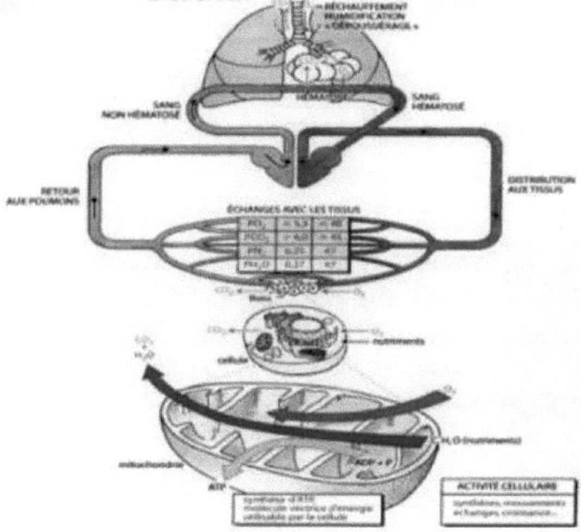

Lung respiration is simply the result of cellular respiration: cells use OO_2 to break down energetic nutrients (e.g. glucose) and produce energy (ATP). This oxidation results in the formation of $CO2$ + H2O.

4.2 Ventilatory mechanics

Ventilation is a periodic phenomenon consisting of a succession of inhalation movements, during which a certain volume of air is inhaled, and exhalation movements, during which a certain volume of air is expelled. These are the processes by which air enters and leaves the lungs.

Gas flows are always established from an area of high pressure to an area of low pressure. Any variation in volume leads to a variation in pressure. The product : P x V = *constant.*

The volume of a gas is inversely proportional to the pressure it is subjected to.

4.2.1 Inspiration: an active phenomenon

Inspiration is an active phenomenon during which thoracic volume increases. On the other hand, alveolar pressure (or lung pressure) decreases. This pressure then becomes lower than atmospheric pressure. This phenomenon therefore allows air (approximately 21% oxygen, 78% nitrogen and a very small amount of CO2) to enter from the mouth into the alveoli. This phenomenon is said to act according to a pressure gradient (i.e. the difference between the pressures inside and outside the lung).

Lung volume is increased by contraction of the inspiratory muscles. These muscles increase the size of the thoracic cavity in all directions (increasing the diameter vertically, transversely and antero-posteriorly).

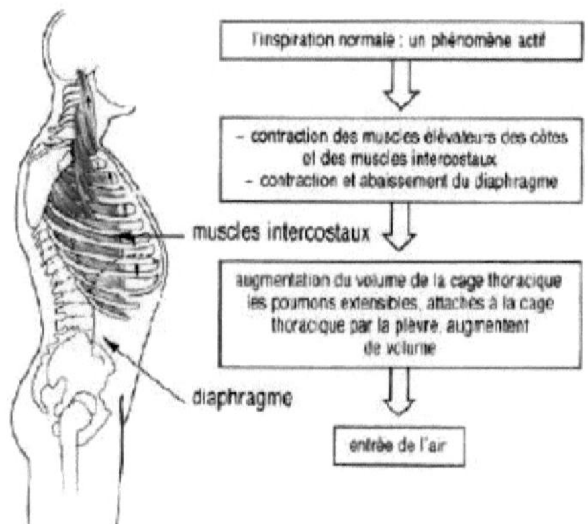

FIGURE 4.2

The main muscle involved in inspiration is the diaphragm. During inspiration, it lowers and pushes the volume of the thoracic cage downwards. It is a flat muscle, known as the radius muscle, which extends between the thorax and the abdomen. It has three fascicles:

- A costal bundle: whose fibres originate from the 7th to 12th cords.

- A vertebral bundle: originating from the lumbar vertebrae.
- A sternal bundle: originating from the xiphoid process.

This muscle has orifices through which vessels pass, including the aorta and vena cava, and

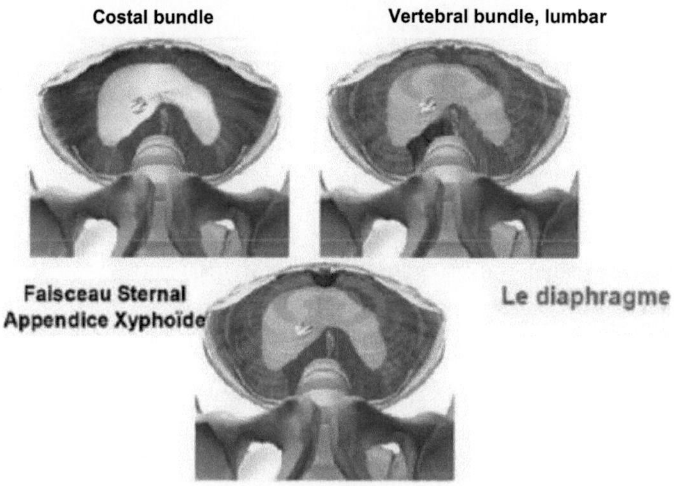

FIGURE 4.3

the oesophagus. This muscle is the main inspiratory muscle.

The external intercostals: these are muscles located between the ribs. They are responsible for outward elevation of the ribs and forward elevation of the sternum.

During forced inspiration, three other muscles are involved:

- **The pectoralis minor:** which originates on the 3rd, 4th and 5th cords and ends on the coracoid process of the ulna.
- **The sterno-cleido-mastoi'dien:** this muscle originates from the occipital line and the mastoi'dien and ends at the level of the sternum and on the medial part of the clavicle.
- **Sealeries:** three in number. They are stretched from the cervical vertebrae to the first two sides.

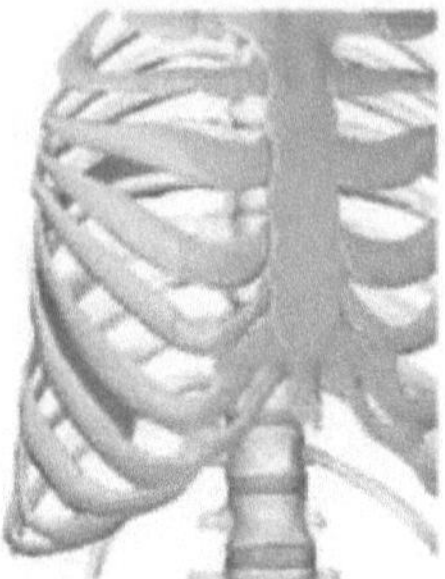

FIGURE 4.4

- **The anterior scalene:** originates at the level of C_3 *a C6* and extends
finishes on the first hill.
- **The middle scalene:** originates from *C? & C7* and ends in
back of the previous one.
- **The posterior scalene:** originates from C_4 a C_6 and ends on the second side.

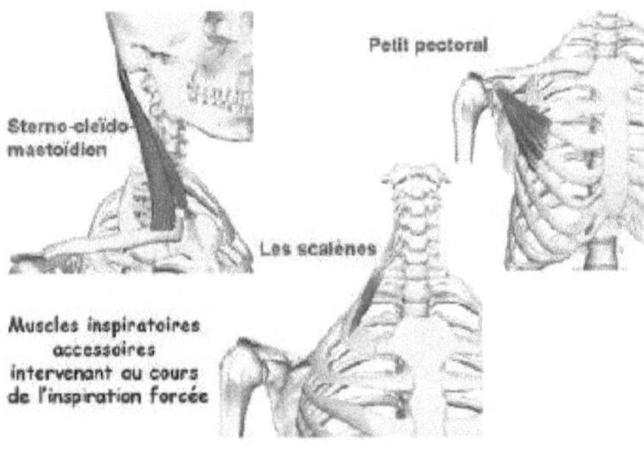

FIGURE 4.5

4.2.2 Expiry: a passive phenomenon

Exhalation is a passive phenomenon that results from the relaxation of the inspiratory muscles and the elastic return of the lung tissue. Stretched during inspiration, the lung then returns to its basic position.

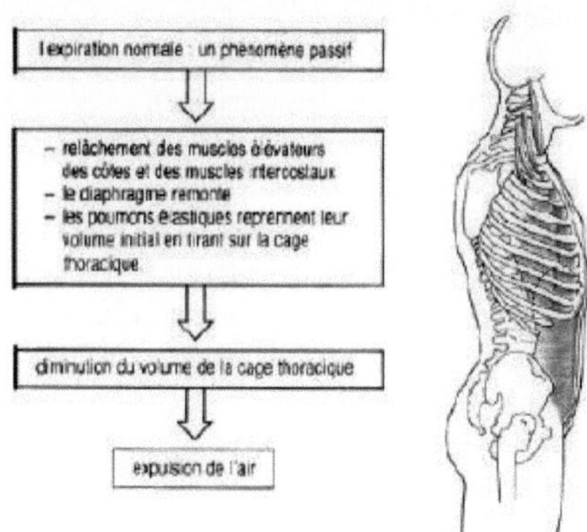

FIGURE 4.6

During exhalation at rest, the relaxation of the inspiratory muscles causes a reduction in the volume inside the lung and therefore an increase in alveolar pressure. This leads to a reduction in the diameter of the lungs and bronchi.

The intra-alveolar pressure will become greater than the atmospheric pressure. This will cause air to escape from the lungs through the pressure gradient.

Forced exhalation is an active phenomenon. It involves the muscles of the abdominal wall, in particular the rectus abdominis and the internal obliques (abdominals). When these muscles contract, they push the diaphragm upwards while the ribs are pushed inwards and downwards. This increases intrapulmonary pressure and decreases volume.

Respiratory muscles active

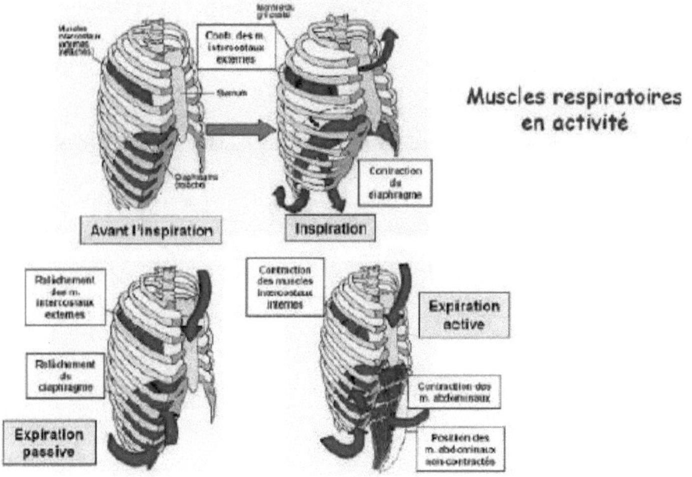

FIGURE 4.7

4.2.3 Breathing volumes

Respiratory volumes (inspiration and expiration) can be measured at rest using what l'on calls

1 functional respiratory exploration (EFR).

EFR is performed using spirometry (volume measurement).
We also define what l'on calls dynamic volumes. Among the dynamic volumes we generally measure the maximum expiratory volume per second (FEV1).
This volume is of little interest on its own. It is related to the vital capacity and the ratio FEV1 / CV (vital capacity) represents the TIFFENEAU index. In all subjects with healthy lungs and green bronchi, Get's index should represent 80% (this means that on exhalation, we should be able to exhale 80% of our vital capacity in the first second of exhalation).
Vital capacity is the sum of three volumes:
- the resting volume known as the tidal volume.
- Inspiratory reserve volume (IRV)
- Expiratory reserve volume (ERV)

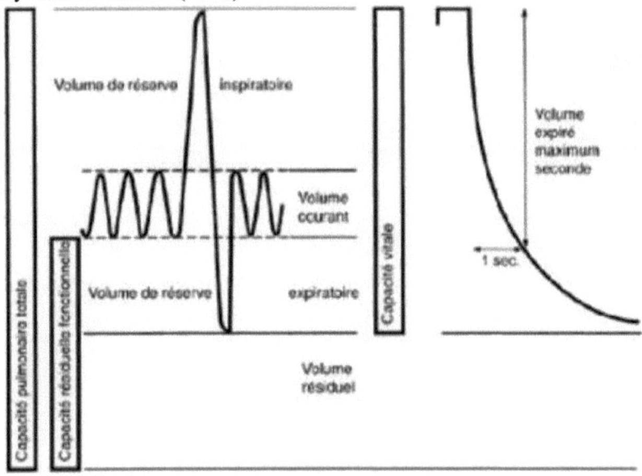

FIGURE 4.8

These volumes depend on age, sex and height. Average values for the different volumes:
- VC = 500 ml
- VRI = 2.5 1
- ERV = 1.5 1
- CV = 4.5 1
- VR = 1 1
- CPT = 5.5 1
- FEV1 = 3.4 1
The spirometer can only measure volumes that can be mobilised (VC, ERV, IRV).

4.3 Gas exchange mechanism

4.3.1 The lungs

The alveolar-capillary wall separates :

- blood from the pulmonary artery (non-hematogenous blood), from
- Γ alveolar air.

Air is a gaseous mixture containing approximately :

Constitution	Air inspires	Air expires
Nitrogen	79% i.e. PN2 = *79KPa*	79% i.e. PN2 = *79KPa*
Dioxygen	20% i.e. PO2 = *20KPa*	15% i.e. PO2 = *15KPa*
Water vapour	0,5%	Saturates
Carbon dioxide	0.04% i.e. *PCO2 = 0.04KPa*	5% i.e. *PCO2 = 5KPa*
Rare gases	Traces	Traces

The pressure of a gaseous mixture such as air is expressed in kiloPascals (kPa). It is equal to the sum of the partial pressures of the different gases, which are proportional to the percentages of the gases in the mixture. *PPN+ + PO2 + PH2O + PCO2)*

The only gases exchanged during respiration are dioxygen and carbon dioxide. Nitrogen is not involved in gas exchange (the level of nitrogen is the same in all compartments).

- The mechanism that causes a gas to move is diffusion.
- The quantity of gas that diffuses is proportional to the difference in partial pressure between the 2 exchange zones and tends towards an equilibrium of the partial pressures between these 2 exchange zones.

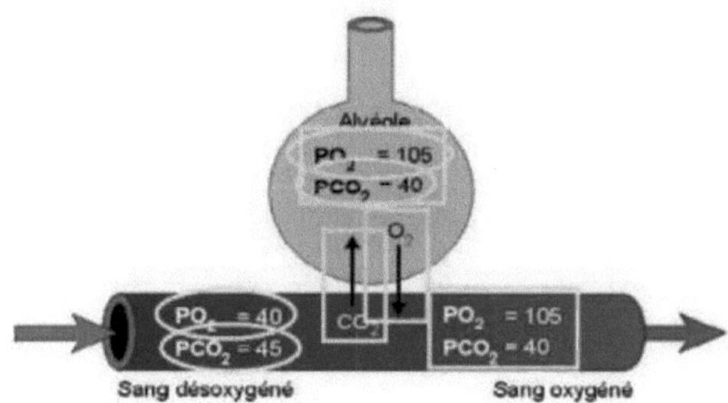

FIGURE 4.9 - Alveolar exchanges

These gas exchanges cause non-hematose blood (or venous blood, dark red) to change into hematose blood (or arterial blood, bright red). Lung breathing causes hematosis: blood entering the lungs is non-hematous and blood leaving the lungs is hematous.

Given the size (600 million pulmonary alveoli and 70m^2 of air-blood contact) and the thinness (about 0.5^m) of the exchange surface, diffusion rates are very fast (diffusion volume *o* 200 to 250 ml per min of resting *O2*).

4.3.2 Tissue level

The thin walls of the capillaries separate the blood from the interstitial lymph, which in turn is separated from the intracellular fluid by the cells' plasma membranes.

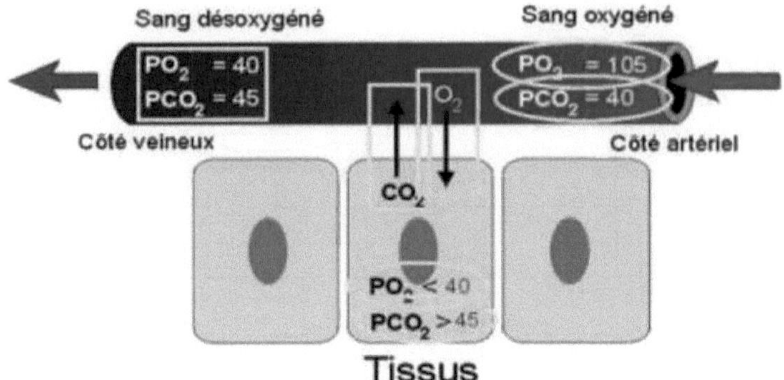

FIGURE 4.10 - At tissue level

Cellular respiration causes the blood to be depleted of O2 and enriched in $CO2$: the blood enters the tissues hematose and leaves them non hematose. The slowness of capillary circulation (= microcirculation) favours the diffusion of gases.

4.3.3 Dioxygen saturation curve for haemoglobin (Barcroft curve)

The percentage saturation of Γ Hb in 02 is the quotient of the rate of oxyhe- moglobin stir l'hemoglobin total.

The O saturation of 1'Hb in O$_2$ as a function of $PO2$ is a sig- moi'de curve which shows that the saturation of 1'Hb in $O2$ increases with $PO2$, but this increase is not proportional.

For low $PO2$ values (from 0 to 2 kPa) or high values (from 8 to 14 kPa) the variation in the % saturation of 1'Hb is low (for example between 8 and 14 kPa: 10 P = 100 - 90). For intermediate $PO2$ values (from 2 to 8 kPa) the variation in the % saturation of 1'Hb is high, i.e. 70% (90 - 20).

The affinity of Hb for O2 molecules varies according to $PO2$:

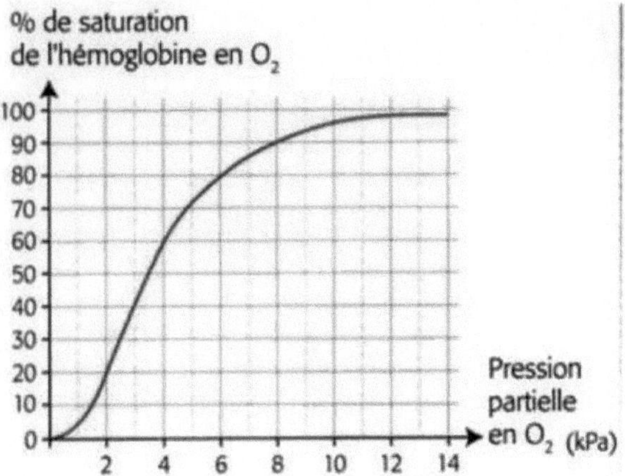

FIGURE 4.11 - Saturation curve

4.3.4 Changes in haemoglobin saturation

1) Effect of CO2

The higher the PCO2, the less O_2 is bound to hemoglobin: the affinity of Hb for O_2 decreases as the *PCO2* increases, and dissociation of oxyhemoglobin is facilitated (the curve shifts to the right).

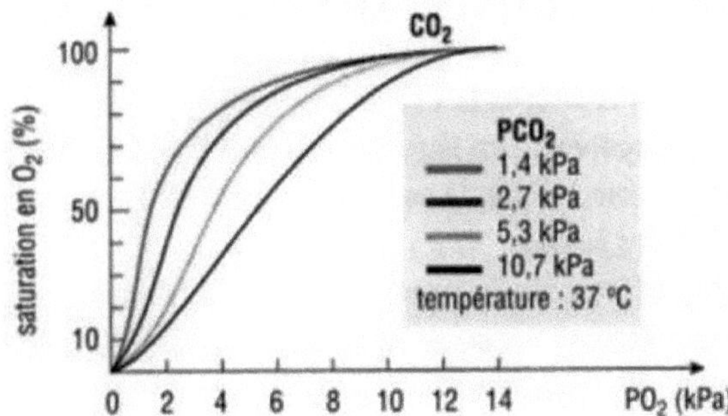

FIGURE 4.12 - Barcroft curve

2) Effect of temperature

The higher the To, the less O_2 is bound to Hb: the affinity of Hb for *O2* decreases as the To increases, facilitating the dissociation of oxyhemoglobin (the curve shifts to the right).

saturation in O_2 (%)

PO_2 in tissue (kPa)

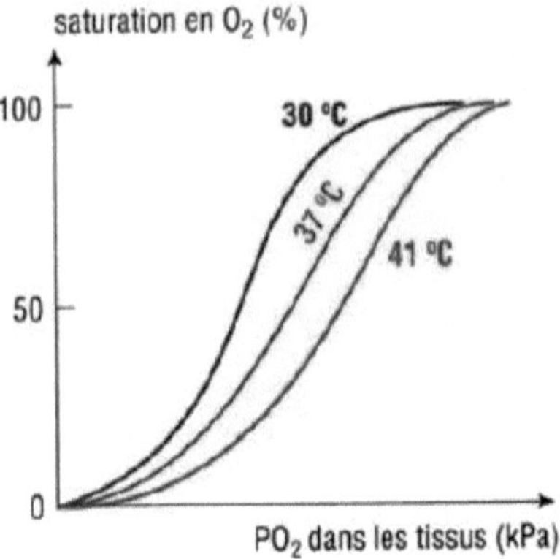

FIGURE 4.13 - Barcroft curve

3) Effect of pH

The lower the pH, the more the curve shifts to the right done there y is less O2 bound to Hb since the % saturation of Hb in O2 decreases: the dissociation of oxyhemoglobin is facilitated.

saturation in O_2 (%)

PO_2 in tissue (kPa)

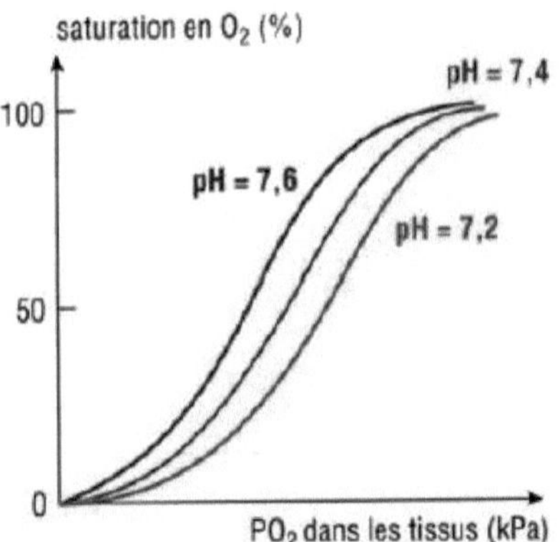

FIGURE 4.14 - Barcroft curve

4.4 Breathing regulation

The main function of the lung is to supply us with 1'02 and to reject *CO2* according to the body's demands in order to maintain a normal level of P_a *O2*, *PaCO2* and pH. There will therefore be a variation, a modification of respiration, which will vary in amplitude and rhythm according to demands.

At rest, we ventilate very little, but during exercise we ventilate more. This is called hyperventilation. This hyperventilation is due to three basic elements that come into play in the regulation of breathing:

- receptors: collect information (=stimuli) and transmit it.
- respiratory centres: these coordinate the information received by the receptors and send impulses to the respiratory muscles.
- The effectors: these are the respiratory muscles (contraction - decontraction - respiration). There is a nervous control of breathing. This nervous control comes from the respiratory centres. There are three respiratory centres (in the brain stem):
- The bulbar centre
- The apneustic centre
- The Pneumotaxic Centre

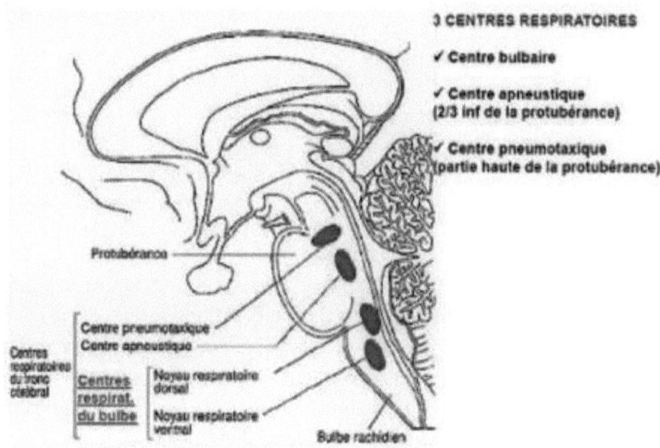

FIGURE 4.15

These three centres define the rhythm and amplitude of breathing by sending nerve impulses to the respiratory muscles. These respiratory muscles are contracted or decontracted by central and humoral stimuli (resulting from chemical modification). There are in fact several modifications that can cause hyperventilation.

4.4.1 Chemical modifications

Any increase in CO_2, any increase in H+ ions and any drop in pH will trigger a command from the central chemoreceptors to the respiratory centres to increase ventilation (to eliminate excess CO_2 and restore pH).

The peripheral chemoreceptors located in the aortic arch and the carotid artery are sensitive to variations in *PO2, PCO2* and pH. In addition, the sensitive fibres from these chemoreceptors are able to transmit the information to the inspiratory centre, which will increase contraction of the diaphragmatic and intercostal muscles (the main breathing muscles) to restore *PCO2* and pH.

In addition to these central and peripheral chemoreceptors, there are mechanical receptors that are sensitive to retirement. These are located in the pleura, bronchioles and alveoli of the lung. These stretch-sensitive receptors stimulate the expiratory centres and cause an increase in breathing. They therefore stimulate the expiratory muscles, which are the abdominal and external intercostal muscles.

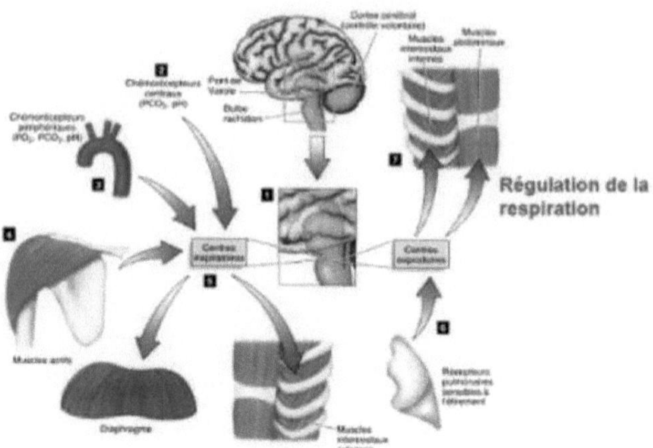

4.4.2 Regulation of breathing during exercise

Breathing can be measured during exercise using a mask connected to oxygen and carbon dioxide analysers. This measures what happens during breathing.

During exercise that progressively increases in intensity, we can see that ventilation initially evolves in a linear fashion, then from a certain intensity onwards, ventilation drops off (this is the first threshold of adaptation of respiration) until a second threshold is reached (the ventilation de-adaptation threshold) where we see ventilation drop off again.

During the first period of effort, ventilation increases in a linear fashion as required. Oxygenation is sufficient and reaches the muscles.

However, from the first detachment, there is an initial increase in acid waste in the blood, an initial increase in the CO2 produced and from SV1 onwards, the intensity is such that blood lactates are first observed (we enter anaerobic metabolism). At this intensity, the quantity of acid waste (H+ ions) is greater and is therefore buffered by the arrival of bicarbonates in the blood.

At the level of SV2, the increase in acid waste and the intensity of exercise is such that bicarbonates are no longer sufficient to buffer lactates and acid waste. There is therefore a sharp increase in H+ ions and therefore a drop in pH, which stimulates the nerve centres and leads to significant hyperventilation.

4.4.3 How does tidal volume and respiratory frequency change?

At rest, the ventilatory rate is around 61 per minute. In fact, the tidal volume is 500 ml and the respiratory frequency is of the order of 12 to 16 respiratory cycles per minute.

During exercise, the ventilatory flow rate increases, firstly by increasing the tidal volume. This tidal volume impinges on the IRV and ERV and then, when the tidal volume can no longer increase, the respiratory frequency increases. The second threshold (SV2) appears when the tidal volume stops increasing. The tidal volume only increases up to 50% of the vital capacity (IRV + ERV + VC).

Training is also an important factor in improving the quality and quantity of breathing. Training improves the number of functional alveoli. The more you train, the greater the surface area for alveolar-capillary exchange. Ventilation is therefore more effective, more profitable and more economical. So you push back the breathlessness threshold.

Chapter 5
Pathophysiology of the respiratory system

5.1 Introduction

Six mechanisms may be involved in the onset of hypoxemia (flashcode 1): reduction in inspired oxygen pressure, true right-to-left shunt, shunt effect due to inadequate ventilation-perfusion ratios, diffusion disorder, alveolar hypoventilation and reduction in oxygen saturation of mixed venous blood.

When the alveolar-capillary oxygen gradient is normal, it can be used to identify isolated alveolar hypoventilation and to guide the etiological diagnosis of hypoxemia, but it requires knowledge of the inspired oxygen fraction (in ambient air or under mechanical ventilation). It increases with age and its normal value can be calculated by the formula: (age in years + 10)/4. When the patient is already undergoing oxygen therapy for ARD, it is dangerous to take a blood gas in air, and its calculation is therefore not required, as follows:

- Alveolar oxygen pressure $PAO2 = (PB - PH2O) \times FiO_2 - PACO2/QR$
- Alveolar-arterial oxygen gradient (D(A-a)02) = PAO2-PaO2

5.2 Impaired pump function

Elie is sometimes primary and linked to a neuromuscular disease (polyradiculoneuritis, myasthenia gravis) and psychotropic drug intoxication (benzodiazepines, barbiturates, etc.).

Elie is often secondary and consecutive to the fatigue of the respiratory muscles caused by the increase in WOB, which the patient cannot cope with completely.

The patient's WOB increases:

- When ventilatory demand is high during hyperthermia or exercise, for example;
- when the compliance of the respiratory system (Crs) is reduced, for example during pneumonia, pulmonary oedema, pleural effusions, pneumothorax under pressure or when the abdomen is distended (abdominal compartment syndrome);
- when airway resistance (Raw) is increased (bronchospasm, bronchial congestion). The increase in Raw can be inspira- tory and/or expiratory;
- when there is dynamic hyperinflation, or trapping, the increase in end-tidal volume generates a residual positive intrathoracic pressure. This positive end-tidal pressure is known as dynamic or intrinsic positive airway pressure (Peep i). The phenomenon of trapping flattens the diaphragm and places it in a geometric structure where its force of contraction is reduced.

The clinical signs of increased WOB are signs of acute respiratory distress: draught, inspiratory depression of the inferior intercostal spaces (Hoover's sign) and the supra-clavicular fossa, thoracoabdominal tilt (the abdomen depresses during inspiration). The onset of respiratory muscle fatigue results in superficial tachypnea: increase in respiratory frequency (RF) and decrease in tidal volume (VT). The increase in fR alters the efficiency of the exchange function by increasing the sweep of areas not involved in gas exchange (dead space: upper airways and large bronchi). Hypoxemia and hypercapnia worsen, and a sometimes mixed ventilatory and metabolic acidosis develops, which also has deleterious effects on diaphragmatic function.

5.3 Impairment of pulmonary exchange function

Impairment of pulmonary exchange function is mainly the result of an alteration in the ratio of alveolar ventilation to pulmonary perfusion (VA/Q), and more rarely of a diffusion disorder. Alteration of the VA/Q ratio results either in an intrapulmonary veno-arterial shunt effect or, on the contrary, a dead space effect.

5.3.1 Intrapulmonary shunt effect

The result is areas with little or no ventilation compared with perfusion. In these areas, ventilation/perfusion ratios (VA/Q) are less than 1, sometimes close to 0. Atelectasis, pneumopathy and pulmonary edema are the main causes of the shunt effect. It is responsible for hypoxemia which cannot, or only partially, be corrected by the administration of oxygen.

5.3.2 Diffusion disorder

It occurs whenever the diffusion capacity of oxygen through the pulmonary interstitium is altered. The main causes of diffusion disorders are interstitial edema, infectious interstitial pneumonia, fibrosis and pulmonary carcinomatosis. Diffusion disorders are usually responsible for hypoxemia without hypercapnia, which can always be corrected by administration of high concentrations of oxygen.

5.3.3 Dead space effect

In contrast to the shunt effect, the dead space effect occurs when a certain number of zones are normally ventilated but not perfused or perfused only slightly. In the dead space effect, VA/Q ratios are greater than 1, and sometimes infinite. Hypertension, heart failure, pulmonary circulation disorders and tachypnea are the main causes of the dead space effect. The dead space effect is responsible for hypercapnia. This can be masked by hyperventilation in response to hypoxemia.

5.3.4 Causes of hypoxemia and hypercapnia

Figure (5.1) shows the different mechanisms that need to be considered to determine the cause of hypoxemia or hypercapnia. This is important because judicious therapy depends on the outcome of the analysis of this mechanism.

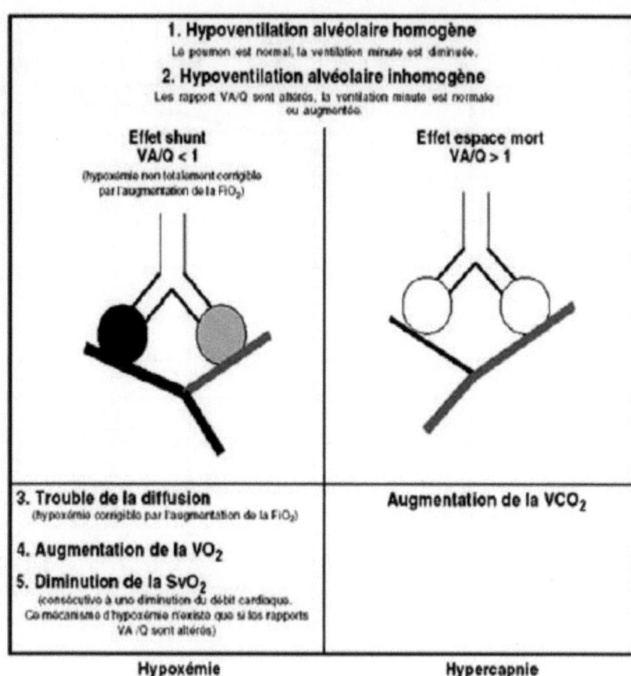

FIGURE 5.1 - Mechanisms of GDS alteration during ARI

It is important to remember that :

- **Homogeneous alveolar hypoventilation** is responsible for proportional hypoxemia and hypercapnia, meaning that the increase in $PaCO_2$ is equal to the decrease in *PaO2*. In the absence of oxygen administration, the sum of *PaCO2 + PaO2* remains close to 140 mmHg. The point representing the relationship between hemoglobin saturation and *PaCO2* on the Sadoul diagram is very precisely on the curve known as homogeneous hypoventilation (Figure 5.2). Homogeneous hypoventilation is the result, for example, of isolated impairment of pump function in neuromuscular disease or psychotropic drug intoxication;

• **in a patient with normal lung exchange function**, significant hypoventilation (< 3 L/min) is required for blood gases to be altered, in particular for PaCO2 to increase significantly;

• **1 inhomogeneous alveolar hypoventilation,** combining the shunt effect and dead space effect to varying degrees, is the most frequent mechanism of GDS al- teration;

• **the decrease in oxygen saturation of the venous mixed blood** (SvO₂) is a frequent cause of worsening hypoxemia when there are alterations in the VA/Q ratios. This is observed when cardiac output decreases while oxygen consumption (VO2) remains constant, or when VO2 increases while Q_c remains constant.

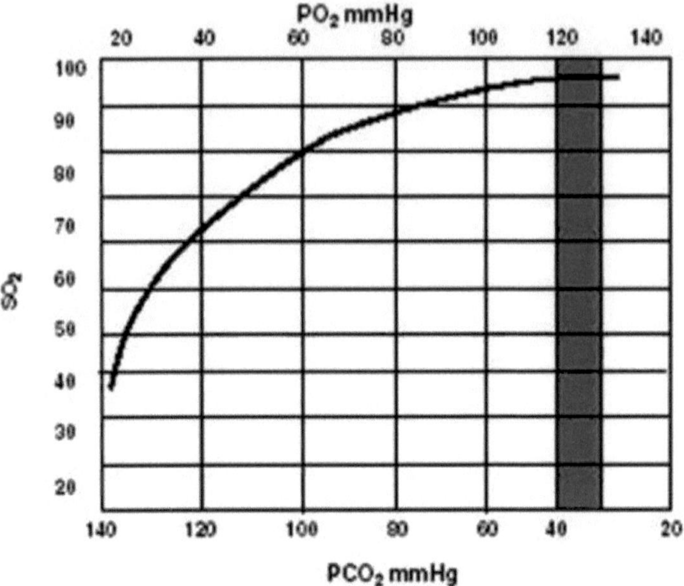

FIGURE 5.2 - Sadoul diagram

Relationship between hemoglobin saturation (SO2) and partial pressure of $CO2$ (PCO$_2$). The curve corresponds to the relationship between these two parameters during homogeneous hypoventilation in a healthy lung (QR = 0.8).

Any deviation from this curve implies therapeutic hyperoxygenation (points above), abnormal ventilation-perfusion ratios (points below) and hyperventilation (points to the right).

5.4 Impairment of transport function and blood analysis

5.4.1 Acid-base balance

It is useful to plot the GDS results on Strihou's Van Ypersele diagram (Figure 5.3). Note that :

• in acute hypercapnia, pH decreases by 0.05 and bicarbonates increase by 1 mEq/L when *PCO2*

• In chronic hypercapnia, bicarbonates increase by 3 to 5 mEq/L when *PCO2*

• to assess the existence of metabolic acidosis associated with acute hypercapnic acidosis, it is simple to calculate the predicted respiratory pH, bearing in mind that a 10 mmHg increase in PCO222

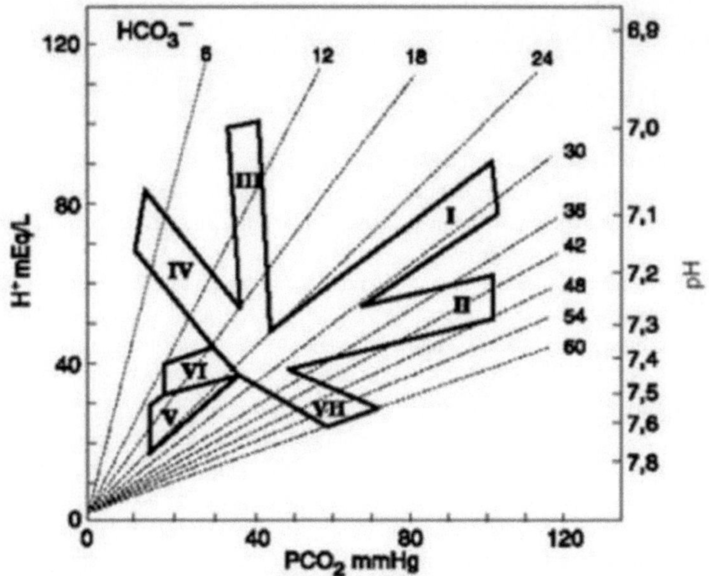

FIGURE 5.3 - Van Ypersele de Strihou diagram (drawing by V. Rolland)

The points included in a zone reflect a simple acute5 acid-base balance anomaly, or a chronic physiologically compensated anomaly. Points outside the zones are outside the confidence intervals and indicate associated disorders.

The concentration of H + ions and the pH are represented on the ordinate, the *PCO2* on the abscissa.

The dotted lines correspond to the concentration of bicarbonate HCO3 in mEq/L. The different surfaces correspond to the buffer zones of plasma in vivo:

- Acute (I) and chronic (II) respiratory acidosis;
- Acute (III) and chronic (IV) metabolic acidosis;
- Acute (V) and chronic (VI) respiratory alkalosis;
- Metabolic alkalosis (VII).

Chapter 6
Ethiologies

6.1 Neuromuscular causes

Neuromuscular diseases can affect tonsillar respiratory muscles, leading to a!§иё respiratory failure (ARF). This is the most frequent cause of morbidity and mortality in these patients. Two situations must be distinguished:

- 1 ARF secondary to acute neuromuscular disease with a reversible component (Guillain-Barre syndrome, myasthenic crisis, etc.).
- ARF occurring in a patient known to have an advanced and possibly progressive neuromuscular disease (amyotrophic lateral sclerosis, Duchenne muscular dystrophy, etc.).

6.1.1 Guillain-Barre syndrome

Guillain-Barre syndrome (GBS), a rare neurological disorder, causes progressive paralysis that starts in the feet and gradually progresses upwards to affect the whole body (ascending paraplegia). It occurs when a person's immune system attacks the body's peripheral nerves. The condition is known as autoimmune and can be triggered by surgery, flu-like illnesses or stomach infections. As the immune system fights the infection, it mistakenly attacks the peripheral nerves.

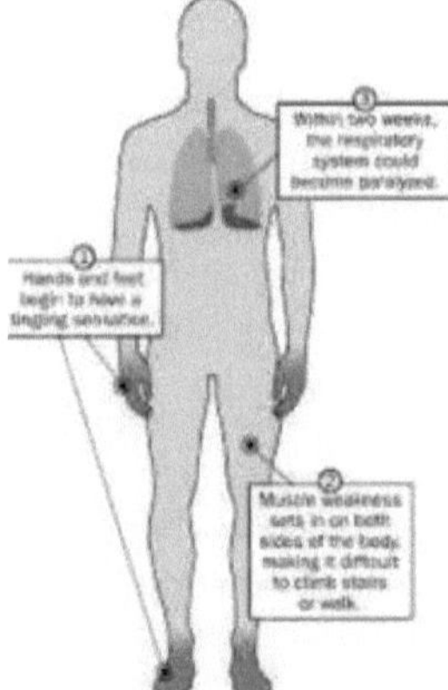

FIGURE 6.1 - Guillain-Barre

GBS affects men and women of all ethnicities and ages. There is a treatment for this syndrome, and 80% of sufferers recover; residual neurological deficit (lasting damage to the nervous system) is nil or minor. The most serious cases require emergency medical treatment, admission to hospital and longer periods of rehabilitation. Approximately 10-15% of sufferers experience residual neurological deficits. These can range from difficulty in running or walking to difficulty in breathing; some people need to use a respirator all the time. Less than 2% of people who contract GBS die from it.

In Guillain-Barre syndrome, the patient's immune system attacks part of the peripheral nervous system. The syndrome affects the nerves that control muscle movement, as well as those that transmit painful, thermal and tactile sensations. This can lead to muscle weakness and loss of sensation in the legs and/or arms.

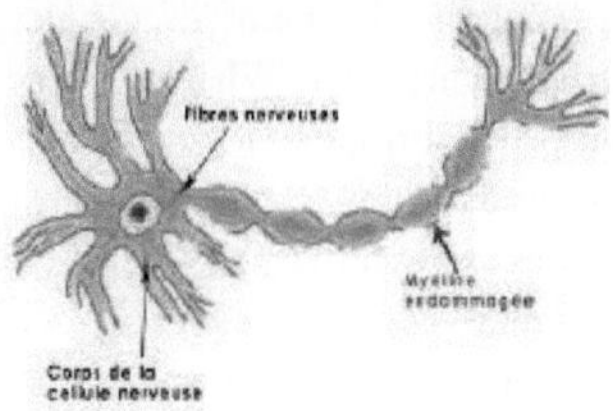

FIGURE 6.2 - Nerve affected by Guillain-Barre syndrome

• The first symptoms of Guillain-Barre syndrome are weakness or tingling, usually starting in the legs and spreading to the arms and face.

• In some patients, these symptoms can progress to paralysis of the legs, arms or facial muscles. In 20% to 30% of patients, the thoracic muscles are affected, making breathing difficult.

• In severe cases, the ability to speak and swallow may be affected; these cases are considered life-threatening and must be treated in intensive care units.

• Most patients make a full recovery, even in the most severe cases, although weakness may persist in some.

• Even in the best healthcare settings, 3% to 5% of patients with Guillain-Barre syndrome develop complications of the disease, such as paralysis of the breathing muscles, sepsis, pulmonary embolism or cardiac arrest.

1) Diagnosis

The diagnosis is based on the symptoms and the results of the neurological examination, in particular the reduction or loss of deep tendon reflexes. A lumbar puncture may be performed to confirm the diagnosis, provided that it does not delay treatment.

2) Treatment

• Guillain-Barre syndrome is potentially fatal. Patients suffering from Guillain-Barre syndrome must be admitted to hospital for close monitoring.

• Supportive care includes monitoring breathing, heart rate and blood pressure. In the event of respiratory compromise, patients generally require assisted ventilation. They must be monitored for possible complications, including abnormal heart rate, infection, thrombosis, hypertension or hypotension.

• There is no cure for Guillain-Barre syndrome, but the therapies available can relieve symptoms and reduce the duration of the disease.

• Due to the autoimmune nature of the disease, the acute phase is usually treated with immunotherapy, either by plasmapheresis to remove antibodies from the blood or by injection of intravenous immunoglobulins. This approach is most often beneficial when initiated 7 to 14 days after the onset of symptoms.

• If muscle weakness persists after the acute phase of the disease, rehabilitation services may be required to help patients regain their muscle strength and ability to move.

6.1.2 Myasthenia gravis

Myasthenia is an autoimmune disorder that affects the point of contact between nerves and muscles. For unknown reasons, the body's immune system, which normally helps to fight infection, attacks the Γ acetylcholine receptors in the muscles.

These receptors normally receive a chemical called acetylcholine, which is released by the nerves at the neuromuscular junction (the point of contact between the nerves and the muscles) and commands muscle contraction. When these receptors are damaged or their function is impaired, the muscles cannot respond to the nerve command and become weaker.

Myasthenia is almost twice as common in women as in men. It most often affects women under 40 and men over 50. However, it can appear at any age. Children are rarely affected. The disease is equally prevalent on all continents. A related condition, congenital myasthenic syndrome, is genetically transmitted. Myasthenic syndrome also probably has a genetic component, but the children of sufferers are only slightly more likely than average to develop an autoimmune disorder.

Myasthenia is a serious condition, but it is generally not fatal. Most people with myasthenia have the same life expectancy as the rest of the population. People with myasthenia gravis experience a reduction in physical activity and quality of life, and more sick days. In severe cases, the chest muscles may weaken to the point where the patient can hardly breathe on their own and may need to be on a ventilator for some time (a few days to a few weeks).

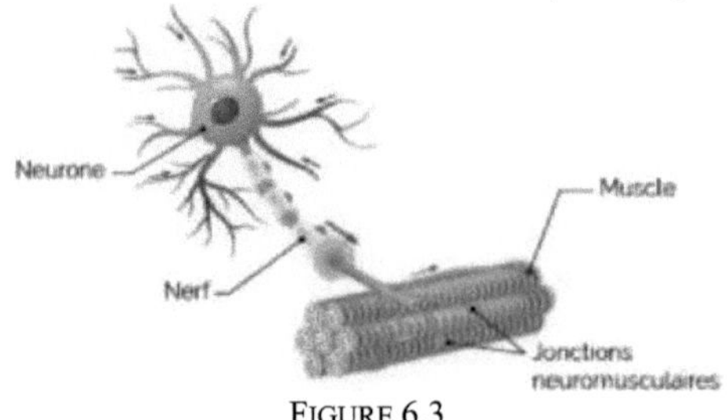

FIGURE 6.3

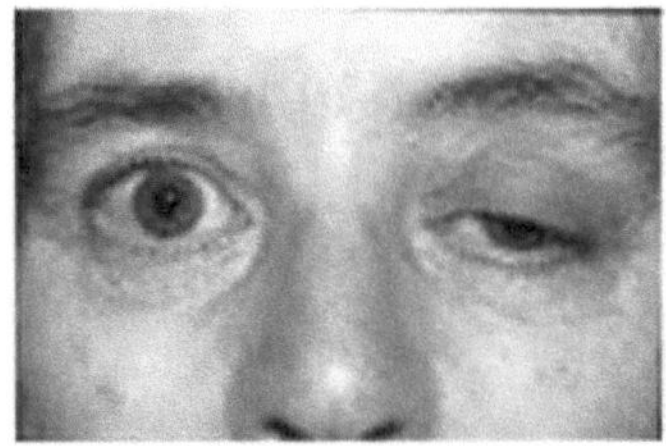

FIGURE 6.4

1) Causes

The exact cause of myasthenia is not known. One theory is that the disease is caused by a virus or other infectious agent with a structure similar to part of the Γ acetylcholine receptor (which Γοπ is found in the neuromuscular junction and which is necessary for it to function properly). The antibodies produced by the immune system to fight the virus then mistakenly attack the receptors.

What we do know is that certain antibodies have been discovered in the blood of people with myasthenia and that they are structured to attack Γ acetylcholine receptors.

In some cases, women with myasthenia pass on these particular antibodies to their babies at the time of birth, resulting in muscle weakness. This is known as neonatal myasthenia and affects around 12% of babies born to mothers with myasthenia. It differs from congenital myasthenia in that the infant's condition improves after a few weeks, as the level of antibodies in the blood decreases.

Some people with myasthenia do not have antibodies against Γ acetylcholine receptors. However, many of them do have antibodies against an enzyme required for the function of the Γ acetylcholine receptor.

The other common abnormality in people with myasthenia is hy- peractivity and excessive size or dysfunction of the thymus gland. The thymus is a gland located at the junction of the neck and chest which is important for the normal development of the immune system. Normally, children are larger than adults, and the thymus becomes inactive at puberty. However, in people with myasthenia, it often remains active into adulthood.

Some people with myasthenia develop thymoma, a tumour of the thymus. This is a type of cancer, but very few people die from it (see the "Treatment and prevention" section).

As well as being caused by infection, symptoms can be triggered by surgery or certain medications.

2) Symptoms and Complications

The most common symptoms of myasthenia are double vision (di- plopia), drooping eyelids (ptosis) and muscle fatigue, which generally worsen after exercise or at the end of the day and improve with rest.

The muscles around the eyes are particularly likely to be affected by myasthenia and visual problems are the first sign of the disease in around 40% of cases. 85% of people with myasthenia eventually develop eye symptoms. Around 15% of people will experience symptoms only around the eyes - these cases are called ocular myasthenias. When symptoms occur elsewhere in the body, they usually do so within 3 years of the onset of ocular symptoms.

Other common symptoms of this disease include:

*   a weakening of the muscles responsible for facial expression;
*   an unstable or unusual approach ;
*   difficulty chewing or swallowing;
*   weakness in the arms, legs, hands and fingers;
*   an inability to stand up without using your hands;
*   blurred vision.

Many subjects experience repeated increases and decreases in the intensity of their symptoms throughout the day. Their symptoms are often the same every day, with maximum muscle fatigue in the evening.

People who are temporarily unable to eat can be admitted to hospital and fed intravenously. A more immediate danger arises when the disease causes respiratory failure. Such episodes, known as myasthenic attacks, are responsible for the rare cases of death caused by myasthenia. People with respiratory problems should go to hospital immediately.

3) The different forms of autoimmune myasthenia gravis

Depending on the distribution of the muscles affected, doctors distinguish between different forms of autoimmune myasthenia:

*   **Ocular myasthenia** is a form of autoimmune myasthenia localised to the muscles of the eyes, which manifests itself by ocular signs: double vision, drooping of one or both upper eyelids... Elie may become genetic in a second stage;
*   **Myasthenia with bulbar involvement,** which affects the muscles of the throat, face, etc., resulting in a face that is not very mobile, a tendency to swallow crookedly, and which is

often generalised in a second stage;

• **Generalized myasthenia** affects all the muscles in the body, in particular the muscles at the base of the limbs: muscles of the shoulders and hips (difficulty lifting the arms, walking, standing for long periods, etc.), neck muscles, muscles used for chewing (tiredness when eating, difficulty closing the mouth, etc.).

The forms of autoimmune myasthenia are also classified according to the antibodies found:

• With anti Γ acetylcholine receptor antibody (anti-RACh),

• With anti-muscle tyrosine kinase receptor antibodies (anti-MuSK), identified around ten years ago, which respond poorly to treatment with anti-cholinesterase agents,

• Double seronegative, i.e. without anti-RACh or anti-MuSK antibodies,

• With anti-LRP4 antibodies (recently discovered).

4) Diagnosis of autoimmune myasthenia gravis

The diversity and variability of manifestations of autoimmune myasthenia means that diagnosis is often delayed, depriving sufferers of effective treatment. In the presence of suggestive signs, the neurologist performs :

• A test consisting of an intravenous injection of prostigmine (or Tensilon®). The disappearance for a few hours of the clinical manifestations and electromyogram signs confirms the diagnosis;

• An immunological test (using a simple blood test) to check for autoantibodies and any associated autoimmune disease;

• A CT scan or MRI of the chest to look for a tumour of the thymus.

5) Treatment

With treatment, autoimmune myasthenia progresses towards stabilisation or even disappearance of the symptoms. The disease fluctuates over time, evolving in flare-ups interspersed with more or less complete remissions. Treatment must therefore be regularly adapted to these fluctuations. Treatment consists essentially of medication and regular monitoring by a specialist consultant.

a) Anticholinesterase agents

Medical treatment is based mainly on anticholinesterase drugs, which inhibit the acetylcholine-degrading enzyme (l'acetylcholi- nesterase), thereby increasing the quantity of acetylcholine at the neuromuscular junction. Mestinon (R), Mytelase (R) and/or Mestinon Retard (R) are the drugs used in doses spread throughout the day.

These products can have sometimes serious side effects: loss of appetite, colic, diarrhoea, salivary and bronchial hypersecretion, slowing of the heart rate (bradycardia). Signs of overdose (muscular fasciculations and cramps, sweating, hypersalivation, bronchial hypersecretion, etc.) should prompt a specialist to be consulted in order to rebalance the treatment.

b) Other treatments

Other treatments are used to reduce the intensity of the immune reaction over time, such as :

• **Corticosteroids** (Cortancyl @, Solupred @);

• **Immunosuppressants** (Imurel (R), Cellcept @);

• **Immunomodulators** (Rituximab);

• **Infusion immunoglobulins,** because plasma exchange has a rapid onset of action;

• **Surgical removal of the thymus** (thymectomy) is often suggested as it appears to improve symptoms over time. It is essential in cases of thymus tumour (thymoma);

6.1.3 Botulism

Botulism is a paralysing disease caused by a toxin (botulinum toxin) produced by a bacterium (Clostridium botulinum). "It's the toxin that makes you sick, not the bacterium itself," explains Christelle Mazuet, head of the National Reference Centre for Anaerobic Bacteria and Botulism at the Institut Pasteur. This toxin is extremely powerful and targets nerve endings. The disease affects both humans and animals, particularly birds and cattle.

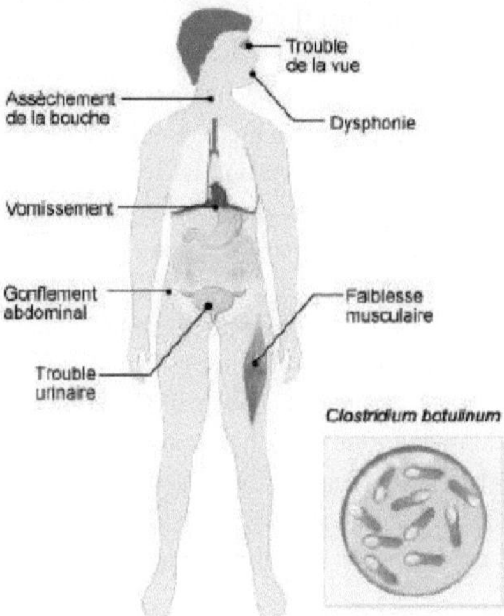

FIGURE 6.5 - Botulism

1) Symptoms

Symptoms usually appear 12 to 36 hours after eating food containing the bacteria and usually last from two hours to 14 days. Symptoms may include nausea, diarrhoea, fatigue, blurred vision, dry mouth, difficulty speaking and swallowing, and descending paralysis extending to the arms, legs, trunk and respiratory muscles. Respiratory failure can lead to death.

2) Causes

The known history of botulism began in 1735, when the disease was associated with the consumption of contaminated sausages and cold meats. The word "botulism" comes from the Latin word for sausage.

There are four main types of this disease: foodborne botulism, infant botulism, intestinal botulism and wound botulism. All forms of this disease can be fatal and should be considered a medical emergency. Foodborne botulism results from the consumption of trans-formed food or drink containing botulinum toxin or spores. It is a rare but potentially fatal condition if not diagnosed and treated promptly. Foods commonly associated with this condition include :

Botulinum toxin has been found in a variety of foods:

- Slightly acid canned vegetables such as green beans, asparagus, beetroot and maize;
- Lightly preserved foods, such as fish, particularly tinned tuna and fermented, dirty or smoked meat.

Wound botulism occurs when spores of Clos- tridum botulinum infect a wound and y produce a toxin. It can result from contamination of a wound by soil, gravel or the injection of illicit drugs.

Infantile botulism affects infants under one year of age and results from ingestion of spores of the Clostridum botulinum bacterium, which germinate in the intestine and produce toxin-releasing bacteria.

Botulism caused by colonisation of the intestine is similar to infantile botulism. It occurs when the C. botulinum bacterium multiplies and produces a toxin in the digestive system. This type of botulism can affect older children and adults who have intestinal problems, such as colitis and intestinal derivation, or other illnesses that can lead to local or general disruption of the normal intestinal flora.

3) Treatment

These food-borne and wound diseases can be treated with antitoxin if diagnosed quickly enough. Antitoxin can stop the disease worsening and reduce the patient's chances of developing complications. Doctors may attempt to remove contaminated food from the patient's digestive system, for example by inducing vomiting. In adults, antibiotics have no effect on botulinum toxin. However, they are necessary for infants in order to destroy the bacteria lodged in the digestive tract.

In cases of severe illness (respiratory failure and paralysis) intensive respiratory care with assisted ventilation may be required for weeks. Serotherapy can also be used, but is only effective if administered within 24 hours of the onset of symptoms.

This pathology, contracted through injury, is often treated by surgical intervention to remove the source of the toxin-producing bacteria.

There is a vaccine, but it is rarely used because it has significant adverse effects. It is reserved for highly exposed people, such as those working in laboratories.

6.1.4 Poisoning

1) Organophosphorus poisoning

Many organophosphorus compounds are powerful nerve agents that act by inhibiting the action of Pacetylcholinesterase in nerve cells. They are one of the most common causes of poisoning worldwide and are often used intentionally for suicide in agricultural areas.

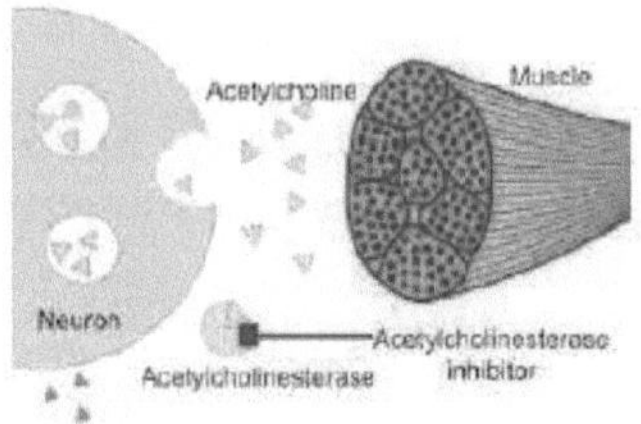

FIGURE 6.6

a) Clinical manifestations :

Classically, three syndromes characterise this type of intoxication.

• Muscarinic syndrome

Muscarinic syndrome associates ocular signs with miosis, accommodation problems, photophobia and ocular pain in the event of direct contact with the eye; respiratory signs with bronchospasm, hypersecretion of the tear, sweat, nose, saliva and bronchi, which can lead to pulmonary oedema; digestive signs with gastrointestinal spasms and colic, faecal incontinence, nausea and vomiting; cardiovascular signs with arterial hypotension due to vasoplegia, bradycardia and then cardiac arrest.

- **Nicotine syndrome**

The nicotine syndrome associates muscular fasciculations and cramps, followed by rapidly increasing asthenia due to damage to the motor plate, evolving towards paralysis of the striated muscles and respiratory arrest. These signs appear later and indicate the seriousness of the intoxication. A my- driasis by excitation of the superior cervical ganglion may be observed, if the toxic agent has not been in contact with the eye. Arterial hypertension with tachycardia may be observed at the onset of intoxication.

- **Central syndrome**

Finally, the central syndrome combines behavioural disorders with ataxia, intense tonic-clonic convulsive seizures and encephalopathy with coma at the same time as respiratory depression. These different symptoms are associated in different ways, depending on the characteristics of the product and the mode of intoxication. These signs are correlated with the degree of decline in AChE and generally appear when the latter falls below 50%; inhibition of more than 90% is the cause of serious intoxication.

b) Treatment

ATROPINE is the antidote for OP intoxication. It acts in competition with acetylcholine at muscarinic receptors, but has no effect on cholinesterases at the neuromuscular junction. It treats bronchospasm and bronchial hypersecretion without combating neuromuscular phenomena.

The dose to be administered depends on the severity of intoxication, the patient's weight and reaction. In general: 2 to 4 mg IV every 10-15 minutes or 0.015-0.05 mg/kg (in children), until signs of atro- pinisation appear (dry mouth, gnawing, tachycardia and mydriasis), and maintain a maintenance dose of 0.02 mg/Kg/hour for 24 hours.

PRALIDOXIME Contrathion® Adults and children over 12: 1 to 2 g by intravenous infusion. It is strongly recommended that pralidoxime is administered slowly. Children under 12 years of age: 20-50 mg/kg (depending on the degree of intoxication) mixed with 100 ml of normal saline and administered by intravenous infusion over 30 minutes. The maximum dose varies from 2 to 12 g per 24 hours. The advantage of these high doses would be to avoid the need for controlled ventilation. However, the side-effects of rapid infusion (500 mg/min) in humans are not negligible and include tachycardia, hypertensive surge, laryngospasm and even neuromuscular block. What's more, the cost of this treatment is high, and its benefits are even questionable in some underdeveloped countries.

Contrathion is a cholinesterase reactivator which acts at several levels in OP intoxication. This product hydrolyses not only the enzyme-inhibitor bond, but also the inhibitor, and acts synergistically with atropine, allowing doses to be reduced. Pralidoxime appears to have an atropine-like effect through interaction with cholinergic receptors, resulting in antimuscarinic, antinicotinic and ganglioplegic effects that increase the anticholinergic potency of atropine fivefold. Pralidoxime is also thought to delay the ageing of the enzyme. However, it must be administered very early otherwise it will be ineffective with neurotoxins, leading to rapid ageing of the enzyme. On the other hand, this product does not cross the hemato-encephalic barrier and is not found in the cepha- lorachidian fluid after parental injection, which makes any central effects questionable despite certain cases of clinical and electroencephalographic improvement under oxime. There is no evidence of a reactivating effect on cerebral cholinesterases.

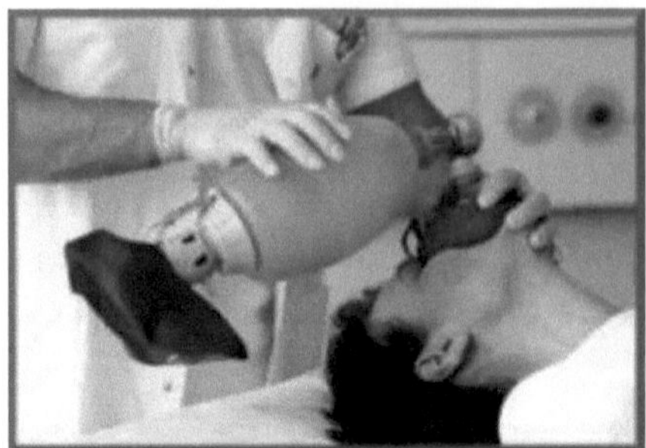

FIGURE 6.7

2) Benzodiazepine poisoning

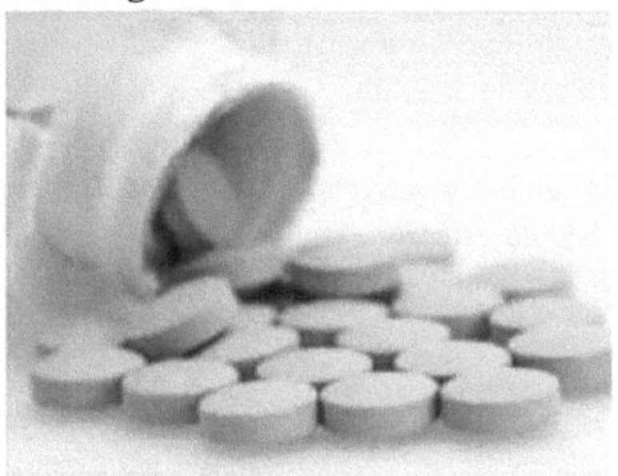

FIGURE 6.8

Benzodiazepines and related molecules have polymorphic properties: anxiolytic, sedative, hypnotic, muscle relaxant and anticonvulsant. The toxidrome is dominated by disorders of vigilance, associated with a myorelaxation syndrome (calm, hypotonic, hyporeflexic coma). Pupils are usually intermediary and reactive, sometimes with mild miosis. Loss of muscle tone in the upper airways leads to increased resistance and obstructive dyspnoea.

As with the majority of psychotropic drugs, the prognosis for benzodiazepine intoxication is usually favourable, and mortality remains low. 11 It is difficult to determine toxic doses for each compound. The greater the quantity of benzodiazepines ingested, the greater the severity of symptoms; but the correlation between suspected ingested doses and symptoms is limited by tolerance phenomena in patients on long-term treatment, and the usual co-ingestion during suicide attempts.

Therapeutic behaviour :

• At infratoxic doses, and in the absence of any signs of seriousness, family surveillance at home is sufficient, with regular water intake recommended, which has no effect on elimination of the product, but has the merit of ensuring that the intoxicated person is still stimulable.

• The benignity of intoxication, when voluntary, does not mean that a subsequent psychiatric consultation is unnecessary

• In the case of a toxic dose or in the presence of signs of seriousness, hospitalisation is necessary with the appropriate resources (SAMU...), depending on the dose, the clinical situation, the time between the intake of the toxic substance and the examination, taking into account the time taken for the plasma peak to appear.

• At l'hdpital

— The value of gastric lavage has not been demonstrated. 11 must be discussed on a case-by-case basis depending on the quantity of toxic substance(s) ingested, the expected toxic effects and the time elapsed since ingestion.

— The clinical benefit of activated charcoal has not been formally demonstrated. It should be administered as a single dose (50 g for adults, 1 g/Kg for children) as soon as possible, at best within 1 hour of ingestion.

— Basic cardioscope

— Intubation and assisted ventilation if justified by the depth of the coma

— Venous hydration without forced diuresis strictly unnecessary

— Neurological and cardiorespiratory monitoring

— Antidotic treatment: flumazenil

6.2 Branchopulmonary causes

6.2.1 Pneumothorax

Pneumothorax is the presence of air in the pleural cavity leading to partial or complete lung collapse. Pneumothorax may be spontaneous or the result of trauma or medical procedures. Diagnosis is based on clinical criteria and chest X-ray. Most pneumothoraxes need to be aspirated or treated by pleural drainage through a thoracostomy tube.

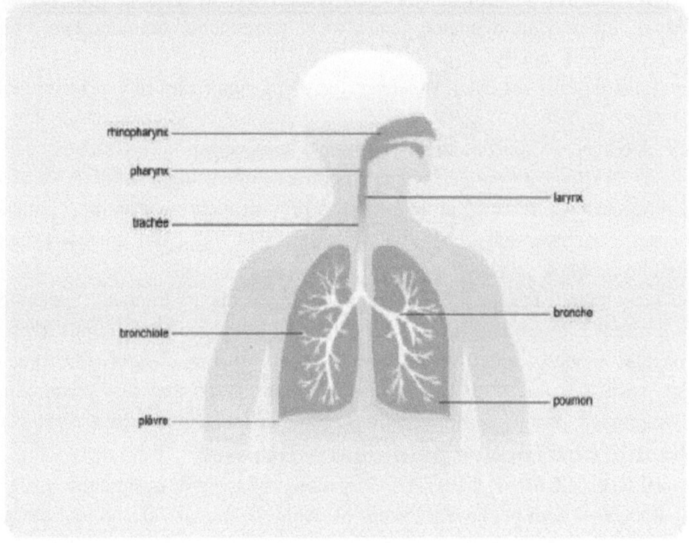

FIGURE 6.9

1) Causes

Primary spontaneous pneumothorax is seen in patients with no underlying lung disease, typically in tall, slim young men between the ages of 10 and 30. It is thought to be due to the spontaneous rupture of apical subpleural bullae or bullae related to smoking or which are congenital. It usually occurs at rest, although some cases occur during activities involving stretching. Primary spontaneous pneumothorax can also occur during pilgrimage and high-altitude flight.

Secondary spontaneous pneumothorax occurs in patients with underlying lung disease. It most commonly results from the rupture of a bulla in patients with severe chronic obstructive pulmonary disease (COPD) (forced expiratory volume in 1 s [FEV1] < 1 L), HIV-associated Pneumocystis jirovecii infection, cystic fibrosis, or other underlying parenchymal lung disease (see table Causes of secondary spontaneous pneumothorax). Secondary spontaneous pneumothorax is more serious than primary spontaneous pneumothorax because it occurs in patients whose underlying lung disease reduces lung reserve.

Catamenial pneumothorax is a rare form of secondary spontaneous pneumothorax which occurs within 48 hours of the onset of menses in non-menopausal women and sometimes in menopausal women treated with oestroge-notreapy. The cause is thoracic endometriosis, probably due to migration of peritoneal endometrial tissue through a diaphragmatic defect or embolisation through pelvic veins.

2) Treatment

Rest, needle aspiration, chest drainage, surgery... Find out about treatments for different types of pneumothorax.

Small, well-tolerated primary spontaneous pneumothoraxes can be treated with rest or exsufllation (evacuation of air) using a needle or small catheter after local anaesthetic. A follow-up X-ray is taken 48 hours later to check that the pneumothorax has resorbed.

The first episode of larger primary spontaneous pneumothorax or one that is poorly tolerated (dyspnea) is treated with placement of a chest tube. Thoracic drainage involves inserting a tube a few millimetres in diameter, under local anaesthetic, between two ribs. If the pneumothorax resolves rapidly

(1 to 5 days), the drain is removed. However, there is a significant risk of recurrence, of the order of 15%.

"Secondary spontaneous pneumothorax requires hospitalisation and emergency pleural drainage," says Dr Clement Fournier. "As the recurrence rate is high, in the region of 40-80%, a surgical procedure is envisaged at the outset to prevent recurrence in most patients, apart from those suffering from cystic fibrosis and awaiting a transplant: pleural symphysis or pleurodesis", he explains.

Drainage is recommended as the first-line treatment for secondary traumatic pneumothorax. It is usually preceded by a chest CT scan to look for associated lesions (hemothorax, tracheobronchial wound, bone fractures, etc.). Two to four weeks after treatment, a consultation with a chest X-ray is recommended to check that the pneumothorax has completely regressed. A number of precautions should be taken to prevent recurrence.

6.2.2 Chronic obstructive pulmonary disease

At respiratory level, COPD is characterised by slow, progressive obstruction of the airways and lungs, associated with permanent distension of the pulmonary alveoli and destruction of the alveolar walls. COPD is characterised by a non-completely reversible reduction in expiratory flow. It is classically associated with chronic bronchitis and pulmonary emphysema.

It is suspected that chronic inflammation of the lungs leads to the muscular dysfunctions observed. In patients with COPD, anaerobic metabolism is used to a greater extent than aerobic metabolism. Overuse of this energy pathway leads to hy- perlactatemia and chronic acidosis. As a knock-on effect, hyperlactatemia will trigger an increase in respiratory frequency and worsen dyspnoe. Maintaining and restoring the functioning of aerobic metabolism now appears to be a major rehabilitation challenge in improving the quality of life of patients suffering from COPD.

The main causes of this disease are smoking (the most common cause)6 and other forms of air pollution11 "the fraction of risk attributable to occupational exposure" has been estimated by epidemiologists at between 15 and 20%. Air pollution is also an aggravating factor, and it would seem that our production model (burning hydrocarbons, pesticides, water pollution, mass diffusion of methane causing the greenhouse effect, etc.) is not going in a direction where COPD could decrease. There are differences and similarities between COPD caused by smoking and COPD caused by work.

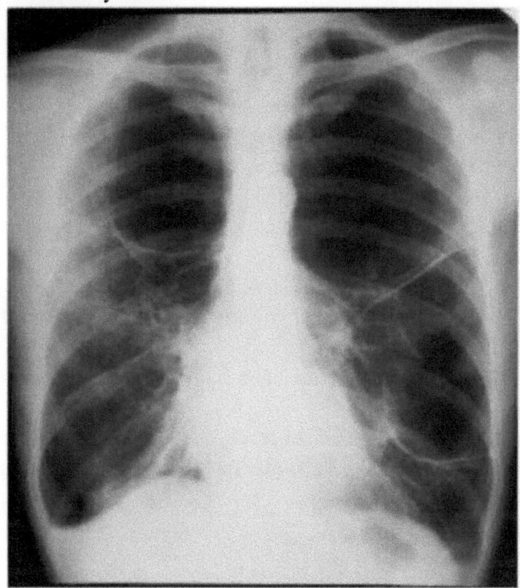

FIGURE 6.10

1) Causes

There are 2 main causes of COPD:

- Smoking (or less often other inhalants)
- Genetic factors

a) Inhalation exposure :

Among exposures to inhaled agents, smoking is the main risk factor in most countries, although only around 15% of smokers develop clinically significant COPD; a smoking history of 40 pack-years or more is an important predictive factor. Smoke from domestic cooking and heating is an important etiological factor in developing countries. Smokers with pre-existing bronchial hyperreactivity (defined as increased sensitivity to inhaled methacholine), even in the absence of clinical signs of asthma, have a higher risk of developing COPD than subjects without bronchial hyperreactivity.

Weight insufficiency, childhood respiratory diseases, passive smoking, air pollution, occupational exposure to dusts (e.g. mineral or cotton dusts) or exposure to inhaled chemical agents (e.g. cadmium) are all risk factors for COPD, but are of minor importance compared with smoking.

b) Genetic factors :

The best defined causative genetic disorder is alpha-l-antitrypsin deficiency, which is a major cause of emphysema in non-smokers and significantly increases susceptibility to the disease in smokers.

More than 30 genetic alleles have been associated with COPD or declining lung function in certain populations, but none has been shown to be as directly involved as Γalpha-l-antitrypsin.

2) Treatment

* Smoking cessation
* Inhaled bronchodilators and/or corticosteroids
* Supportive care (e.g. oxygen therapy, respiratory rehabilitation)

The management of COPD includes the treatment of chronic disease in a stable state and the treatment and prevention of exacerbations. The treatment of chronic lung cancer, a frequent complication of severe long-term COPD, is covered elsewhere.

Smoking cessation is an essential part of COPD treatment.

Treatment of chronic stable COPD is aimed at preventing exacerbations and improving lung and physical function. Symptoms should be relieved rapidly, mainly with short-acting beta-adrenergic drugs, and exacerbations reduced with inhaled corticosteroids, long-acting beta-adrenergic drugs, long-acting anticholinergic drugs, or a combination of these (see table Initial treatment of COPD).

Pulmonary rehabilitation includes structured and supervised exercise, nutritional advice and self-management education.

Oxygen therapy is indicated in selected patients. The treatment of exacerbations consists of ensuring sufficient oxygenation and a blood pH close to normal, removing airway obstruction and treating any underlying causes.

6.2.3 Severe acute asthma

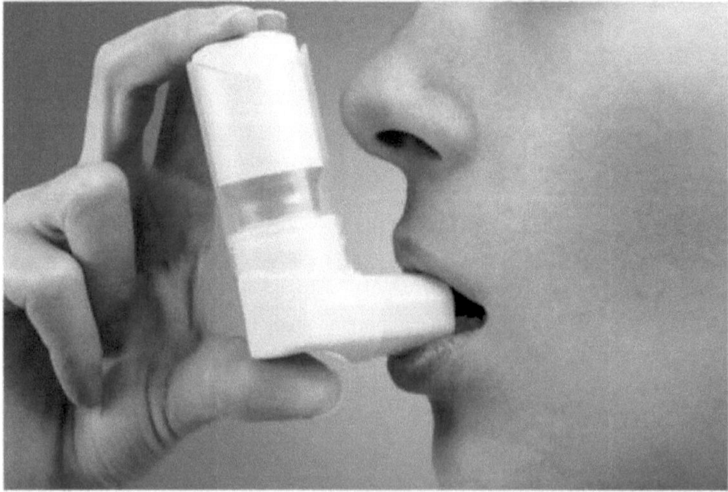

FIGURE 6.11

Acute asthma (or "asthma attack") is a common reason for consultation in emergency departments, and can be associated with a life-threatening risk, as well as significant costs. Effective management of acute asthma involves recognising and assessing the severity of the attack, treating it, deciding whether or not to admit the patient to hospital, deciding whether or not to admit the patient to intensive care and, when the patient returns home, preventing an early recurrence.

Moderate acute asthma (MAA)	• Increase in symptoms • FP >50 • No history of severe acute asthma
Severe acute asthma (SAA)	> one of the following points: • 30-50% PF • EN>25 • FC *110 • Incapacitfc 1 hire a sentence in one breath
Severe acute asthma (life-threatening asthma)	*one of the following: Clinic Measurements • Unconsciousness - FP <30 • Respiratory exhaustion - SpO_2 < 92 • Arrhythmia-PaO_2 < 8 kPa • Hypotension-$PaCO_2$ • Cyanosis4 .5-6 kPa • Absence or- FR > 30/min j sibilance- HR > 120/min • Dyspnea between words
Asthma with imminent respiratory arrest	• Confusion, drowsiness • Breathing break • PCO_2 >6 and/or mechanical ventilation required • Bradycardia. Hypotension • Auscultatory silence

FIGURE 6.12 - Assessment of the severity of acute asthma

1) Causes

The AAG can be called in most cases. It is consecutive to :

• an exacerbation of chronic asthma, usually at night;

• a viral illness, such as winter colds and bronchitis;

• physical effort ;

where it is triggered unexpectedly by :

• an allergy - food allergy or airborne allergy (pollen, animal hair, dust, etc.);

• in the presence of an irritant or toxic substance in Fair (pollution, solvents);

• following a state of intense stress, such as a psychological shock or night-time anxiety.

It can occur gradually or suddenly. Elie requires emergency treatment followed by immediate hospitalisation.

2) Treatment

AAG requires emergency treatment with salbutamol or F adrenaline.

a) Salbutamol :

It is a fast-acting bronchodilator that dilates the small bronchial tubes, allowing Fair to circulate. This medicine has changed the lives of many asthmatics since 1969, when it was developed by Sir David Jack.

There is salbutamol:

• in gaseous aerosol, requiring hand/lung coordination (emptying the lungs, pressing down and breathing in at the same time);

• in powder aerosol, without coordination (activate mechanism, empty lungs, inhale);

43

- nebulised (administered at Fhopital).

b) Adrenalin :

This is a solution that is injected into the thigh muscle. It comes in the form of a self-triggering pen (Epipen®). In Fhopital, it is injected intravenously.

You should always carry your emergency treatment with you and know how to use it.

During hospitalisation, other treatments are added, such as Foxygeno-therapy.

c) Oxygen therapy

It must be treated as quickly as possible, which is why you should not hesitate to go to emergency or call the emergency services.

6.3 Thoracic flap

The thoracic flap or costal flap is a type of rib fracture involving at least three adjacent ribs, each with at least two fractures (i.e. six fractures in total). This type of fracture occurs after a high-energy accident. One of the symptoms is paradoxical breathing.

6.3.1 Diagnosis

Its definition is the existence of at least 2 costal fracture sites over 3 storeys (i.e. a minimum of 6 fracture sites, and 3 broken ribs in 2 portions).

The flaps can be anterior (the mobile segment includes the sternum), lateral (the mobile segment consists solely of ribs) or posterior (which are more stable thanks to the muscle masses).

For the anterior flap, it is accepted that the fracture sites involve the costal cartilages or even the sternum.

The lateral flaps cause the flap to breathe paradoxically, contrary to the respiratory movements (it comes out a Γ expiration and goes in on inspiration).

All of these lesions are seen in high-energy accidents, such as road traffic accidents. These fractures are very painful (due to direct lesions or hematoma close to the intercostal nerves) and this pain also has a negative impact on ventilatory function.

As the triggering mechanism is quite violent, lesions of the thoracic contents are often associated. Numerous complications are possible: pneumothorax (due to penetration of the costal fragment into the pleura), hemothorax and hemopneumothorax (due to embrochage of the intercostal vessels), pulmonary lacerations and contusions. Lung contusions and traumatic pleural effusions are the most common.

X-rays can only partially assess the flaps, and it is often the thoracic CT scan that provides an accurate assessment of the lesions. Ultrasound of polytrauma (FAST ultrasound) can detect pneumothorax, hemothorax and, with greater ease, areas of alveolar condensation due to contusion.

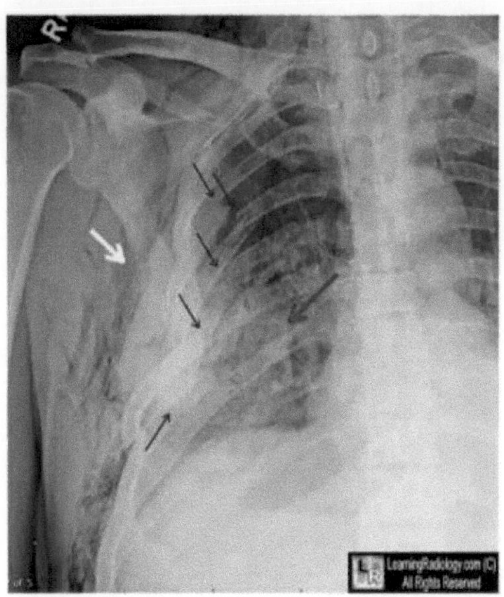

FIGURE 6.13

6.3.2 Treatment

The treatment for a simple rib fracture is pain relief (prescription of painkillers). This treatment can last up to one or two months, depending on the individual.

Management of complicated fractures requires treatment of the complication in addition to pain relief. In general, simply placing a drain in the pleural space (which can be done under local anaesthetic in the patient's bed) will resolve the problem in a few days. However, in some cases, surgery may be required.

The thoracic flap poses a more complex problem. Treatment requires intubation and prolonged assisted ventilation (i.e. the patient's breathing is ensured by a machine). In well-selected cases, surgical stabilisation (i.e. fixation of the various sites of costal fracture by plates screwed to the sides during an operation) may make it possible to avoid this long stay in intensive care and mechanical ventilation.

Patients with thoracic trauma usually undergo a chest X-ray. The purpose of this examination is to visualise the rib fracture(s), if possible. However, this examination is mainly carried out to rule out the presence of a complication. A pneumothorax may be minor and require no treatment, or in some cases it may be life-threatening.

If, with each breath, a little more air enters the pleural cavity than can escape, a tension pneumothorax is formed, compressing and deforming the large venous structures inside the thorax and preventing the return of blood to the heart. The patient's life is at risk if the pneumothorax is not drained immediately. Similarly, a hemothorax may be of lesser importance, or it may represent a significant loss of blood, also threatening the patient's life.

6.4   Bronchopulmonary tumours

Most often, the diagnosis of bronchopulmonary cancer is made when respiratory symptoms (cough, dyspnoea, hemoptysis, etc.) are present or persist, particularly in smokers or former smokers. But the absence of risk factors, the main one being active or passive smoking, does not rule out the possibility of the disease. Other signs may be revealing, in particular extra-pulmonary symptoms associated with metastasis (cerebral, bone, liver) or a paraneoplastic syndrome. It may also be discovered by chance on imaging carried out for another indication.

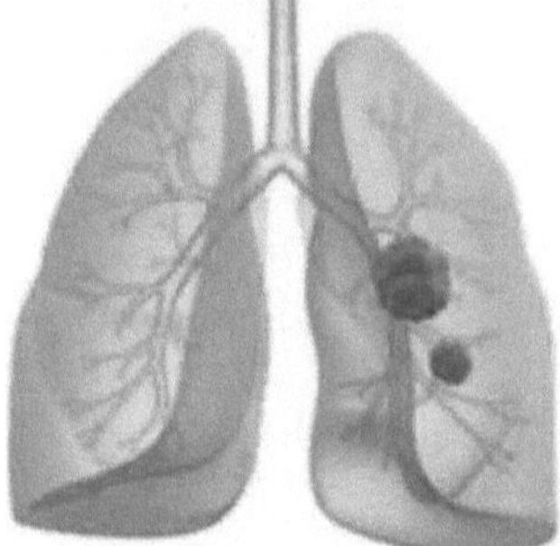

FIGURE 6.14

6.4.1 Treatment

Small-cell lung cancer is a therapeutic emergency.

The therapeutic approach to small cell lung cancer is based on :

•   raclio-chemotherapy, for forms localised to the thorax and accessible to the same radiotherapy field;

•   or exclusive chemotherapy for other forms.

Surgery is reserved for very specific cases.

In addition, prophylactic cerebral irradiation is indicated for patients in complete remission.

6.5   Cardiovascular causes

6.5.1 Acute lung oedema

Classically, there are two types of PAO: cardiogenic or hydrostatic pulmonary oedema and lesional pulmonary oedema, also known as acute respiratory distress syndrome in adults. This chapter will focus on cardiogenic PAO.

Fluid movement within the lung is determined by Starling's law: the net transvascular flow rate depends on the membrane's coefficient of permeability, the hydrostatic pressure between the microvessels and the perivascular interstitium, and the difference in oncotic pressure between the general circulation and the perivascular space. The filter fluid is low in proteins, which are blocked by the interstitium of the pulmonary capillaries.

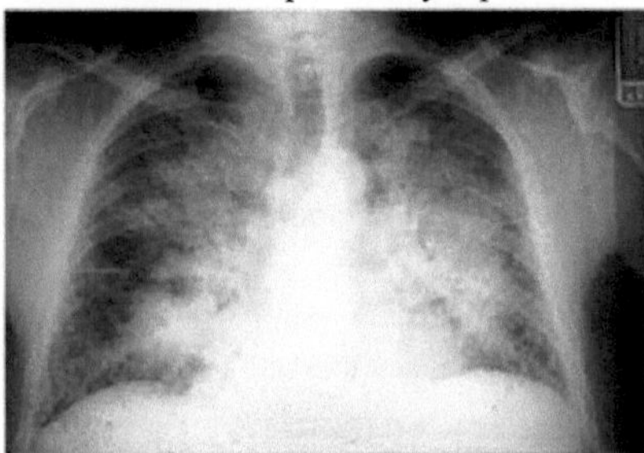

FIGURE 6.15

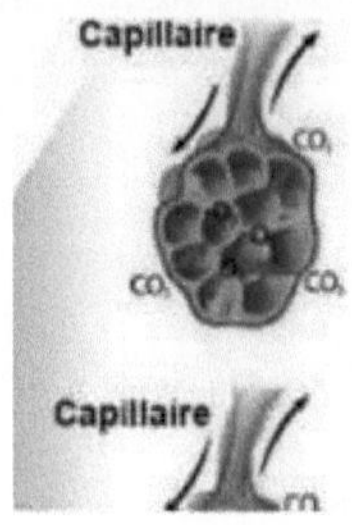

FIGURE 6.16

1) Symptoms

PAO can occur gradually, worsening gradually or suddenly. In its early stages, pulmonary oedema leads to :

- an intense dry cough (sometimes a hacking cough);
- sometimes pink frothy sputum (characteristic of OAP);
- severe shortness of breath, a source of anxiety;
- difficulty breathing and speaking when lying down;
- an increase in pulse and blood pressure;
- cyanosis (bluish discolouration of the lips due to poor oxygenation of the tissues).

When pulmonary edema results in severe respiratory failure, it is a medical emergency, as the patient is at risk of dying from asphyxia.

2) Treatment

If acute pulmonary edema is an emergency (in the event of respiratory distress, exhaustion, signs of shock, etc.), EMS intervention is necessary. The emergency teams will organise rapid revascularisation, reassess the diagnosis and transfer the patient to the emergency department or even to a cardiac intensive care unit.

The patient must remain seated (head and chest elevated) and we proceed :

- oxygenation, or even assisted ventilation via intubation in severe cases;
- a l administration of medicines :
- diuretics (by infusion, then orally) to eliminate water from the lungs,
- vasodilators (depending on the level of blood pressure),
- anticoagulants,
- tranquillisers if the patient is particularly anxious.

With appropriate management, PAO can be cured within a few hours. However, 50% of patients suffer recurrences within 12 months. Of course, finding and treating the cause is essential.

In extreme cases, a heart transplant may be considered.

6.5.2 Pulmonary embolism

Pulmonary embolism is the blockage of a pulmonary artery or one of its branches, usually by a blood clot. It causes damage to the affected lung, and the lesioned part can no longer supply oxygen to the body.

The clot forms during venous phlebitis or thrombosis (usually in the legs). It detaches from the wall of the vein and rises with the blood in the venous circulation towards the heart. During its contractions, the heart's right ventricle propels the clot into the pulmonary arteries.

The blood clot travels through increasingly narrow arteries, where it eventually becomes blocked.

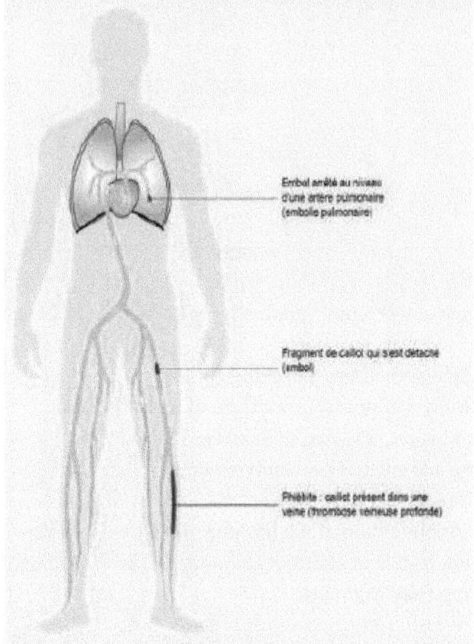

FIGURE 6.17

1) Symptoms

Pulmonary embolism causes a sudden onset of :
- chest pain on one side, which increases on inspiration;
- difficulty breathing (dyspnoea): rapid, short breathing;
- sometimes a cough and sputum with blood.

Symptoms are sometimes difficult to identify because they are not very intense or specific. Difficulty in breathing may occur gradually, and pain may be moderate.

Symptoms vary from one person a Γ another, but they should always raise a red flag when they occur in a context where there is a risk of phlebitis and pulmonary embolism (following surgery, immobilisation in the previous month, cancer undergoing treatment...).

Other symptoms may be present, often in cases of severe pulmonary embolism:
- feeling unwell, or even losing consciousness;
- an increase in heart rate (tachycardia);
- low blood pressure ;
- peripheral signs of shock (mottled knees, blue fingers and lips, cold hands and feet).

2) Treatment

Treatment of pulmonary embolism depends on its severity and the patient's condition.
- Pulmonary embolism: essential anticoagulant treatment
- Thrombolysis of the clot
- Surgical embolectomy and catheter-directed thrombolysis

48

Chapter 7
Additional examinations

Measurements of physiological constants (heart and respiratory rates, blood pressure, oxygen saturation) complete the clinical examination and allow a rapid assessment of the seriousness of the situation. Few additional tests are needed to establish the diagnosis of respiratory distress9. In an emergency, chest X-rays and arterial blood gases are the only tests required to make the diagnosis^. Depending on the initial indications, other tests may be carried out to determine the cause of respiratory distress. However, these should not delay the start of treatment.

The standard blood test may point to a cause: hyperleukocytosis in the case of bacterial infection, elevated CRP in the case of inflammation, increased D-dimer in the case of pulmonary embolism, increased BNP in the case of cardiac failure.

Cardiac and pleural ultrasound can be useful in differentiating the causes of hypoxemic respiratory failure. Chest computed tomography (CT) can be used to look for pulmonary embolism or signs of fibrosis, or to clarify lesions seen on the chest X-ray. In the event of infection (fever or purulent sputum), sputum analysis and blood cultures can be used to identify the causative organisms. In febrile patients, influenza is systematically investigated during epidemics.

Bronchial fibroscopy may be indicated when the cause of respiratory distress is not obvious5. It allows bacteriological samples to be taken, as well as exploring the morphology of the bronchial tree by taking biopsies if necessary, and performing bronchoalveolar lavage.

7.1 Measuring arterial blood gases :

Gasometry consists of measuring the oxygen and carbon dioxide content of the blood contained in the arteries in order to identify any abnormalities in the distribution of these gases, which are essential for the body to function properly. In the event of respiratory insufficiency, blood gas measurement reveals :

- hypoxemia, in other words a lack of oxygen in the blood.
- hypercapnia, i.e. an overload of carbon dioxide in the blood, if the disease is at a more advanced stage.

7.1.1 Performing an arterial blood gas test

Arterial gasometry is used to analyse acid-base balance (pH) and measure arterial oxygen pressure (PaO2) and arterial carbon dioxide pressure (PaCO2). It can also be used to determine a patient's respiratory status.

This test is indicated for any severe respiratory condition or suspected major metabolic disorder. It can help to make a diagnosis, guide therapy and assess its effectiveness, but it also has prognostic value. It is therefore important to remember to check the results of this test and to communicate them to the doctor as soon as possible.

The patient is first informed of the treatment we are going to perform. The patient's pulse is checked, an Allen test is carried out and an anaesthetic patch is applied if possible.

a) Preparing the equipment

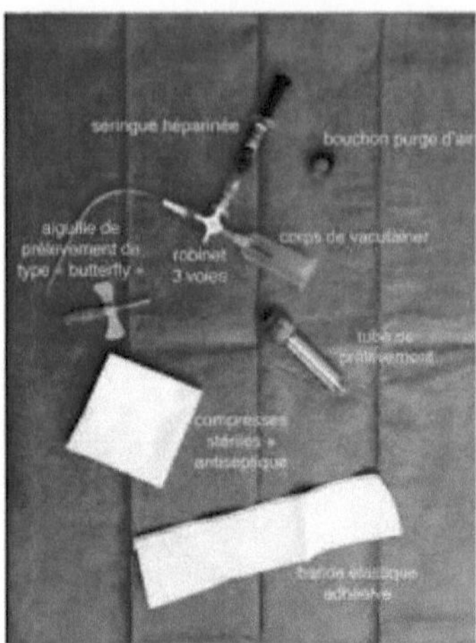

FIGURE 7.1 - Blood gas equipment and sampling.

- a care trolley with a DASRI bag, a DAOMI bag and a needle box;
- a hydro-alcoholic solution;
- a pair of non-sterile gloves;
- a specific syringe (heparin) with a safety needle;
- compresses;
- an antiseptic;
- plasters.

In the event of an additional deduction, you will also have to :

- a vacutainer with an adapter;
- a butterfly needle;
- a 3-way valve ;
- sample tubes as prescribed by the doctor.

b) Procedure

- Perform the Allen test, if it has not already been carried out.
- Check the medical prescription and the patient's identity (surname, first name and date of birth).
- If the patient is on 02, the doctor may ask for the examination to be carried out in room air, in which case 1'02 must be removed 10 minutes before the sample is taken.
- Take the patient's temperature and oxygen saturation (necessary for the laboratory to read the results).
- Set up ergonomically.
- Using your index and middle fingers, locate the patient's artery at wrist level in extension: you should feel the blood pulsating through your two fingers.
- Prepare the equipment. If additional sampling is required, adapt the ring on one port of the tap, the adapter on the other and the butterfly needle on the third port, otherwise use a needle from the specific gas syringe.
- Disinfect your hands and put on gloves.
- Disinfect the puncture site using compresses soaked in antiseptic.
- Prick the artery until the bright red blood pulsates into the syringe. Puncture with the

50

butterfly needle, tap open towards the syringe. When the pre-heparinised syringe is at least 1 mL full, turn the tap and fit the collection tubes. Unlike venipuncture, a blood gas syringe is not under vacuum. The blood fills the syringe under l'effect of pulsatile arterial pressure.

• Remove the syringe and compress the puncture site for 5 minutes before applying a plaster dressing.
• If the patient is conscious, tell them how important it is to report the appearance of any abnormal signs such as pain, hematoma, sensation of paralysis, etc.
• Seal the syringe, expel the air bubble and sort your waste before closing the bin liners. Remove your gloves.
• Reposition the patient if necessary.
• Promptly dispatch the syringe labelled with the patient's name, together with the completed application form.

c) Normal values

Analyse	Valeur normale	Unité
pH	7,38–7,42	
PaCO$_2$	38–42	mmHg
PaO$_2$	> 90 selon l'âge	mmHg
HCO$_3^-$	23–27	Mmol/L

FIGURE 7.2 - Normal values

d) Analysis

As a reminder, the pH is kept stable by the joint action of the lung (which controls *PaCO2)* and the kidney (which controls the production of bicarbonates, HCO3-):

$$pH = constante + \log \frac{HCO_3^-}{PaCO_2}$$

This formula shows that the pH is constant if the ratio $HCO_3^- / PaCO_2$ remains stable.

There are several important questions to ask when analysing a blood gas result:
• Is there a pH imbalance?
• When the pH is altered, is the disorder metabolic or respiratory?
• Is this disorder compensated?

pH	PaCO$_2$	HCO$_3^-$	Résultat	Étiologies
N	↑	↑	Acidose respiratoire compensée	Insuffisance respiratoire chronique
↓	↑	N ou ↑	Acidose respiratoire non compensée	Hypoventilation alvéolaire : – insuffisance respiratoire aiguë – décompensation de BPCO
↓	N ou ↓	↓	Acidose métabolique non compensée	Acidocétose Acidose lactique (hypoxie) Insuffisance rénale
↑	N ou ↓	↑	Alcalose métabolique non compensée	Vomissement ou aspiration digestive par sonde nasogastrique Traitement diurétique
↑	↓	N ou ↓	Alcalose respiratoire non compensée	Hyperventilation alvéolaire sur poumon normal : – effet « blouse blanche », angoisse – effet physique Hyperventilation alvéolaire induite par une hypoxémie (stade précoce) : – OAP – embolie pulmonaire – pneumonie, bronchite et crise d'asthme non grave

FIGURE 7.3 - Interpretation of a blood gas

7.2 Functional respiratory examination (FRE) and spirometry

Functional respiratory testing (FRT) is used to assess the severity of respiratory insufficiency by measuring respiratory capacity using various parameters: total pulmonary capacity (TPC), forced expiratory volume in one second (FEV1) and vital capacity (VC). Functional respiratory investigation (FRI) is also used to identify the cause of respiratory failure, which may be obstructive, restrictive or mixed.

Lung function tests (LFTs) are carried out by a lung specialist, either in hospital or in the community. This examination is based mainly on spirometry, a functional respiratory exploration test that assesses lung function. Sitting with your nose blocked by a clamp, you blow as fast and as hard as you can through a mouthpiece connected to a spirometer, which in turn is connected to an electronic measuring device. The data collected during spirometry is then compared with that of an individual with normal respiratory capacity.

7.2.1 Examination principles

Functional respiratory examinations (FRE) are a series of tests used to assess respiratory capacity.

• **Spirometry is** used to study ventilation rates (in particular FEV1: forced expiratory volume in one second, i.e. the maximum volume that the patient can exhale in one second) and mobilisable volumes (vital capacity: total volume mobilised after maximum inspiration and expiration). It is used to diagnose bronchial obstruction (e.g. asthma, COPD). It is the basic EFR test.

• **Plethysmography** measures all lung volumes, including residual volume (i.e. the volume of air remaining in the lungs after maximum exhalation). Get exam is carried out in a closed cabin in which the patient sits on a seat. Plethysmography is used to diagnose a restrictive syndrome (diffuse interstitial lung disease, pulmonary fibrosis, cypho-scoliosis, etc.) or thoracic distension (emphysema).

- **Pulmonary diffusion capacity is** used to assess the transfer of oxygen from the pulmonary alveoli to the blood vessels. Measuring diffusion is useful in cases of emphysema, interstitial pathology or fibrosis and pulmonary arterial hypertension (PAH).

- **Arterial gasometry** (measurement of blood gases) is a blood puncture in the artery (and not in the vein like conventional blood tests). It is used to determine the oxygen (pO2) and carbon dioxide (pCO2) pressure in the arterial blood.

- **Other specific tests** may be requested by the respirologist, such as measurement of pulmonary resistance, a metacholine challenge test (to detect bronchial hyper-reactivity), measurement of respiratory muscle power (Plmax, PEmax and SNIP test), or a hyperoxia test (to look for a shunt).

7.2.2 Who should take the test?

These examinations are useful in a great many situations in pneumology, in particular for :

diagnosis and monitoring of chronic respiratory diseases (chronic obstructive pulmonary disease (COPD), emphysema, asthma, etc.)

- assessment before lung surgery (thoracic surgery in particular) or certain other operations that may have consequences for breathing

- monitoring of certain diseases that affect the respiratory system (cystic fibrosis, sclerodermia, etc.)

- monitoring respiratory function in patients treated with drugs that can cause respiratory complications (methotrexate, bleomycin, etc.)

7.2.3 How is the examination conducted?

Spirometry, plethysmography and diffusion capacity measurements are painless tests in which the patient is asked to breathe into a mouthpiece. A nose clip is also used to avoid distorting the measurements.

Different manoeuvres are carried out: first the patient breathes slowly, then he is asked to inhale and then exhale as far as possible. These exercises are repeated 2 or 3 times (sometimes more) to ensure they are reproducible. These tests last between 15 and 45 minutes. They are completely painless. In some cases, the patient may be placed in a small cabin with transpa- rent walls for a few minutes to carry out these exercises.

Gasometry involves drawing blood from the radial artery (wrist). Pain may be felt during the puncture. This blood test takes just a few minutes. To prevent the formation of a hematoma, a compression bandage is applied to the wrist after the procedure. This must be kept on for at least 20 minutes.

7.3   Lung imaging

Doctors can rely on two imaging tests: X-rays and chest CT scans. They are not essential, but they provide images of the lungs and airways, and of the interactions between the two, and can help to identify the cause of respiratory insufficiency.

Thoracic imaging includes unprepared X-ray, computed tomography, magnetic resonance imaging (MRI), scintigraphy, positron emission tomography (PET) and ultrasound.

There are no absolute contraindications to non-invasive imaging procedures except for FIRM. The presence of metal objects in the patient's eye or brain prohibits FIRM.

The presence of a permanent pacemaker or internal defibrillator is a relative contraindication (see MRI Safety). In addition, gadolinium, when used as a contrast agent for FIRM, increases the risk of systemic nephrogenic fibrosis in patients with stage 4 or 5 chronic kidney disease or those on dialysis. Gadolinium may be harmful to the foetus and is generally avoided during pregnancy.

7.3.1 X-ray techniques

X-ray techniques used to image the thorax include

- Rx without preparation
- Radioscopy
- High-resolution spiral CT scan
- Angio-CT

a) Rx thorax

Chest X-ray and fluoroscopy are used to provide images of the lungs and surrounding structures.

Chest x-rays provide images of the structures in and around the thorax, and enable abnormalities of the heart, lung parenchyma, pleura, chest wall, diaphragm, mediastinum and hilum to be identified. They usually constitute the initial examination carried out to assess the lungs.

The standard chest X-ray is taken from the back to the front (frontal view) to minimise scattered X-rays, which could artificially widen the cardiac silhouette, and from one side of the chest (lateral view). Dynamic extension (lordotic) or oblique views can be taken to assess pulmonary nodules or to analyse abnormalities linked to superimposed structures, although CT of the chest provides more information and has largely superseded this type of view. Lateral decubitus views can be used to distinguish free pleural effusion from compartmentalized pleural effusion, but CT or Doppler CT are not suitable for this purpose.

Ultrasound can also provide further information. End-expiratory films can be used to detect small pneumothoraxes.

Screening chest x-rays are often carried out but are almost never indicated, with the exception of asymptomatic patients with a positive tuberculin intradermo-reaction, in whom a single frontal chest x-ray without a prohl film can be used to decide on further diagnostic tests and/or treatment for pulmonary tuberculosis. Chest x-rays performed with portable machines (usually with a frontal click) are rarely of optimal quality and should only be performed when the patient cannot be transported to the radiology department.

Radioscopy of the thorax involves using a continuous beam of x-rays to visualise movements. It is useful for detecting unilateral diaphragmatic paralysis. During a "sniff test", the patient inhales forcibly through the nose ("sniff"). If a hemidiaphragm is paralysed, it moves upwards (paradoxically), whereas the normal hemidiaphragm moves downwards.

b) Computed tomography (CT)

CT shows intrathoracic structures and abnormalities with greater precision than the chest x-ray. Conventional (planar) CT provides multiple images of the thorax in 10 mm thick cross-sections. Its main advantage is that it is widely used. The disadvantages are movement-related artefacts and limitations on the volume of tissue within each 10 mm slice.

Thoracic CT is normally performed with full inspiration. Ventilation of the lungs during imaging provides the best views of the lung parenchyma, airways, vasculature, and abnormal signs such as masses, inhltrates, or fibrosis.

High-resolution CT provides slices 1 mm thick. High-resolution CT is particularly useful for assessing the following disorders

- Interstitial lung diseases (e.g. carcinomatous lymphangitis, sarcoidosis, idiopathic pulmonary fibrosis [hbrosing alveolitis])

- Bronchiectasis

High-resolution CT scans of complete expiration and inspiration may be useful. Expiratory imaging can document Lair trapping, which is a hallmark of bronchiolitis obliterans and other airway diseases. Supine images can differentiate between dependent atelectasis (which changes with changes in body position) due to lung disorders that cause glass-stack attenuation of the posterior dependent parts of the lungs, which persists despite changes in patient position (e.g. fibrosis due to idiopathic pulmonary fibrosis, asbestosis, or scleroderma).

Helical (spiral) CT provides multiplanar images of the entire thorax while the patient is in apnea for 8 to 10 seconds while being moved through the machine. Helical CT is considered to be at least equivalent to conventional CT in most indications. Its main advantages are its speed, lower exposure to radiation and the ability to reconstruct images in 3 dimensions. The software can also produce images of the bronchial mucosa (virtual bronchoscopy). Its main drawbacks are its limited availability and the need to hold one's breath during the examination, which can be difficult in cases of symptomatic lung pathology. The new multidetector (multi-slice) CT technology enables faster digitisation of the entire thorax, and provides high-resolution thin-slice imaging.

CT angiography uses a bolus of IV contrast to highlight the pulmonary arteries, which is useful in the diagnosis of pulmonary embolism. The contrast load is comparable to that of conventional angiography, but the examination is faster and less invasive. Several studies have confirmed the ability of CT angiography to detect pulmonary embolism, so that it has largely replaced conventional lung scintigraphy and ventilation/perfusion testing (except in cases of intolerance to contrast products).

7.3.2 Nuclear magnetic resonance imaging (MRI)

MRI has a relatively limited role in lung imaging, but is preferred to CT in specific circumstances, such as the assessment of

- Tumours of the superior scissure
- Possible cysts
- Cpii lesions affecting the chest wall

If pulmonary embolism is suspected and IV contrast cannot be used, MRI can sometimes identify a large proximal embolism, but it often has limitations in this condition.

Its advantages are the absence of radiation exposure, excellent visualisation of vascular structures, absence of bone artefact and excellent soft tissue contrast.

The disadvantages are airway and cardiac movements, the duration of the procedure, the cofits associated with FIRM and the occasional presence of contraindications, which include many imaging devices and certain metallic foreign bodies. Gadolinium contrast can be harmful to the foetus, so the use of contrast is generally avoided during pregnancy.

7.3.3 Ultrasound

Ultrasound is often used to facilitate procedures such as pleural puncture and central pulmonary artery catheterisation.

Ultrasound is also very useful for assessing the presence and size of pleural effusions and is now commonly used at the patient's bedside to guide thoracentesis. Bedside ultrasound can be used to diagnose pneumothorax and is increasingly used as an extension of the clinical examination.

Endobronchial ultrasound is increasingly used in conjunction with bronchoscopy to localise masses and enlarged lymph nodes. The diagnostic yield of transbronchial lymph node aspiration is higher with endobronchial ultrasound than with conventional unguided techniques.

7.3.4 Scintigraphy

Scintigraphic imaging techniques of the thorax include

- Ventilation/perfusion (V/Q) scintigraphy

Positron emission tomography (PET)

a) Ventilation/perfusion scintigraphy

Ventilation/perfusion scintigraphy uses inhaled radioisotopes to assess ventilation and IV radioisotopes to assess perfusion. Areas of non-perfused ventilation, non-perfused perfusion or apparent increases and decreases can be detected by 6 to 8 cliches of the lung.

Ventilation/perfusion scintigraphy is most often used in the diagnosis of pulmonary embolism, but has largely been replaced by CT angiography. However, ventilation/perfusion scintigraphy is still indicated in the diagnostic evaluation of pulmonary hypertension in chronic thromboembolism.

Split-function ventilation scintigraphy, in which ventilation is quantified for each lobe, is used to predict the effect of lobe or lung resection on respiratory function; the post-surgical forced expiratory volume in 1 s (FEV1) is estimated by the percentage of tracer uptake in the same fraction of the lung multiplied by the pre-operative FEV1 (in litres). A value < 0.8 L (or < 40% of the patient's theoretical value) indicates limited lung reserves and an unacceptably high risk of peri-operative morbidity and mortality.

b) Positron emission tomography (PET)

PET uses labelled glucose (fluorodeoxyglucose) to measure metabolic activity in tissues. It is used in pulmonary disorders to determine

- If pulmonary nodules or mediastinal lymph nodes harbour the tumour (metabolic stage)
- If the cancer recurs in previously irradiated scarred areas of the lung

PET is more effective than CT in assessing mediastinal extension because it can identify tumours in normal-sized lymph nodes and in extra-thoracic sites, avoiding the need for invasive procedures such as mediastinoscopy or needle biopsy.

The current spatial resolution of PET is 7 to 8 mm; the test is useless for lesions < 1 cm. PET detects metastases in up to 14% of patients in whom they would not previously have been suspected. The sensitivity of PET (80-95%) is comparable to that of histological examination of tissues. False-positive results may occur in the presence of inflammatory lesions such as granulomas. Slow-growing tumours (e.g. bronchoalveolar carcinoma, carcinoid tumour, some metastatic cancers) may cause false-negative results.

New combined CT-PETs are routinely used for the diagnosis and staging of lung cancer.

7.4 Complete cardiological examination

The heart is examined using an electrocardiogram and cardiac ultrasound; the aim is to look for pulmonary arterial hypertension linked to hypoxemia (reduced oxygenation of arterial blood) and signs of right heart failure, a consequence of chronic respiratory insufficiency.

A complete general examination is essential to detect the periphe- rial and systemic effects of heart disease and the existence of ex- tracardiac disease that may affect the heart. The clinical examination includes :

- Measuring vital parameters
- Palpation of the pulse and auscultation
- Observing the veins
- Thoracic inspection and palpation
- Cardiac percussion, palpation and auscultation
- Lung examination, including percussion, palpation and auscultation
- Examination of the abdomen and limbs

Cardiac auscultation is dealt with in a separate section. Despite the ever-increasing use of cardiac imaging, auscultation at the patient's bedside remains useful because it is always available and can be repeated as often as desired, free of charge.

The examination also includes the collection of other patient data.

7.4.1 Vital signs

Vital signs include

- Blood pressure
- Heart rate and rhythm
- Breathing frequency
- Temperature

Additional data often obtained with vital signs include patient weight and peripheral oxygen saturation (SpO2).

Blood pressure is measured on each arm and, if congenital heart disease or peripheral vascular disease is suspected, on both legs. The inflatable part of a well-fitted cuff covers 80% of the circumference of the limb and 40% of its length. The first sound heard when the cuff is decompressed indicates systolic pressure; the disappearance of the sound corresponds to diastolic pressure (5th phase of Korotkoff's sounds). A pressure difference of up to 15 mmHg between the right and left arms is normal; a greater difference suggests a vascular anomaly (e.g. dissection of the thoracic aorta) or a peripheral vascular disorder. Leg pressure is usually 20 mmHg higher than arm pressure. To obtain an accurate blood pressure reading, the patient should

- Sitting in a chair (not on the examination table) for > 5 minutes, with your feet on the floor and your back supported.
- The limb must be worn and held at heart level with no clothing covering the area where the cuff is fitted.
- Refrain from exercising, drinking caffeine or smoking for at least 30 minutes before the measurement is taken.

Cardiac frequency and rhythm are assessed by palpation of the carotid or radial pulses, or by cardiac auscultation if rhythm disorders are suspected; certain beats during rhythm disorders may be audible but may not produce a palpable pulse.

An abnormal respiratory rate may indicate cardiac decompensation or primary pulmonary disease. Heart rate increases in heart failure or anxiety and decreases or becomes intermittent in moribund patients. Rapid shallow breathing may indicate pleural pain.

The temperature may rise during rheumatic fever or a heart infection (e.g. endocarditis).

After a myocardial infarction, low-grade fever is very common. Other causes are only investigated if the fever persists for more than 72 hours.

Weight is measured at each clinical visit with the patient standing and, ideally, wearing a similar amount of clothing. In heart failure, weight gain may indicate hypervolemic disease, whereas weight loss may indicate cardiac cachexia (unintentional non-edematous weight loss >5% in the last 12 months, 1). A history and additional Γ clinical examination results (jugular veins, lung and extremity examinations) are required to determine whether weight changes are related to changes in muscle or fat volume and/or quantity.

Peripheral arterial oxygen saturation (SpO2) is measured. Pulse oximetry measures the oxygen saturation of haemoglobin in arterial blood (SpO2) and provides a rapid, non-invasive estimate of tissue oxygenation. Pulse oximetry is obtained using a probe attached to a finger or earlobe. The general consensus is that *SpO2* 95% is normal, while values < 95% suggest hypoxemia. A notable exception to this threshold value is chronic obstructive pulmonary disease; in these patients, the target *SpO2* is 88-92%. Potential causes of hypoxemia include pulmonary oedema in patients with heart failure and right-to-left intracardiac shunts (patent foramen ovale in pulmonary hypertension, congenital heart disease including tetralogy of Fallot).

a) Ankle-arm index

The ankle-arm index is the ratio of systolic arterial pressure at the ankle to that at the arm. When the patient is lying down, ankle blood pressure is measured at both the dorsal and posterior tibial arteries and brachial blood pressure is measured at both arms at the brachial artery. The index is calculated for each lower limb by dividing the highest pressure of the dorsal artery of the foot or posterior tibial artery at that extremity by the highest of the 2 systolic pressures of the brachial artery. This ratio is usually > 1. A Doppler probe can be used to measure ankle arterial pressure if pedal pulses are not available. easily palpable.

A low ankle-arm index (< 0.90) indicates peripheral arteriopathy which may be classified as mild (0.71 to 0.90), moderate (0.41 to 0.70), or severe (< 0.40). A high index (> 1.30) may indicate that the leg vessels are non-compressible, as can occur in conditions associated with calcification of blood vessels, e.g. diabetes, end-stage renal disease and Monckeberg arteriosclerosis. A high index may suggest that other vascular tests are required (toe-arm index or arterial duplex tests).

b) Orthostatic changes

Blood pressure and heart rate are measured in the supine, sitting and standing positions, with an interval of one minute between each change of position. A difference in blood pressure of *<10mmHg* and a change in heart rate of <20 beats per minute are normal; the difference in blood pressure tends to be somewhat greater in the elderly due to loss of vascular elasticity.

c) Paradoxical pulse

Normally during inspiration, the decrease in systolic blood pressure can be as much as 10 mmHg and the pulse increases to compensate. An exaggeration of this normal response with a greater decrease in systolic blood pressure or a weakening of the pulse during inspiration is considered a paradoxical pulse. The paradoxical pulse is observed in

- Cardiac tamponade (frequently)
- Constrictive pericarditis, severe asthma and sometimes chronic obstructive pulmonary disease

- Restrictive cardiomyopathy, severe pulmonary embolism or hypovolemic shock (rare)

Arterial pressure falls during inspiration because negative intrathoracic pressure increases venous return and fills the right ventricle; as a result, the interventricular septum bulges slightly into the left ventricular outflow chamber, reducing cardiac output and thus BP. This mechanism (and the drop in systolic blood pressure) is exaggerated in diseases that cause high negative intrathoracic pressure (e.g. asthma) or restrict right ventricular filling (e.g. cardiac tamponade, cardiomyopathy) or blood flow (e.g. pulmonary embolism).

The paradoxical pulse is quantified by inflating the cuff just above systolic arterial pressure and deflating it very slowly (e.g. < 2 mmHg/beat). The pressure corresponding to the first audible Korotkoff sounds is noted (initially, only during Γ expiration) and then when they become permanent. The difference between the pressures represents the "quantity" of paradoxical pulse.

7.4.2 Pulse

a) Peripheral pulses

The main peripheral pulses of the arms and legs are palpated for symmetry and volume (intensity). The elasticity of the arterial wall is noted. Absence of pulses suggests arteriopathy (e.g. atherosclerosis) or systemic embolism. Peripheral pulses may be difficult to palpate in obese or muscular patients. In diseases with rapid arterial circulation (e.g. arteriovenous septal defect, aortic insufficiency), the pulse rises rapidly and then collapses. The pulse is rapid and racing in hyperthyroidism and hypermetabolic states; it is slow and sluggish in hypothyroidism. If the pulses are asymmetric, auscultation of the peripheral vessels may detect a murmur due to stenosis.

b) Carotid pulses

Observation, palpation and auscultation of the two carotid pulses may suggest a specific disorder (see table Carotid pulse amplitude and associated disorders). Ageing and arteriosclerosis lead to stiffening of the vessels, which tends to mask the characteristic signs. In very young children, the carotid pulse may be normal, even in the presence of severe aortic narrowing.

Auscultation of the carotid arteries helps to differentiate between murmurs and superadded noises. Heart murmurs originate from the heart or large vessels and are usually most prominent above the superior precordial region, fading towards the neck. Vascular murmurs, which are more acute, are heard only in the arteries and appear more superficial. A distinction must be made between arterial murmurs and venous murmurs. Unlike the arterial murmur, the venous "hum" is usually continuous, best heard when the patient is sitting or standing, and disappears on compression of the homolateral internal jugular vein.

7.4.3 Veins

a) Peripheral veins

The peripheral veins are examined for varicositis, arteriovenous malformations and shunts, and for inflammation and pain on palpation due to thrombophlebitis. An arteriovenous malformation or shunt is indicated (on auscultation) by a continuous murmur, and often, on palpation, by a thrill (because, in systole and diastole, resistances are always lower in the veins than in the arteries).

b) Neck veins

Examination of the neck veins enables the height and shape of the venous pulse to be assessed. The height is proportional to right atrial pressure, while the shape of the wave reflects the events of the cardiac cycle; both are best observed at the level of the internal jugular vein.

The jugular veins are usually examined with the patient seated at 45°. The sonimeter of the venous pulse is normally just above the clavicles (normal upper limit: 4 cm above the sternal fork in the vertical plane). The venous pulse is elevated in heart failure, vascular overload, cardiac tamponade, constrictive pericarditis, tricuspid narrowing, obstruction of the superior vena cava or reduced compliance of the right ventricle. In severe cases, the venous pulse may extend as far as the jaw, and its peak can only be detected when the patient is sitting upright or standing. The venous pulse is weak in cases of hypovolemia.

Normally, the venous pulse can be briefly increased by firm hand pressure on the abdomen (hepatojugular or abdominojugular reflux); this increase disappears in a few seconds (maximum 3 respiratory cycles or 15 s) despite pressure on the abdomen (because a compliant right ventricle increases its stroke volume according to the Frank-Starling mechanism). However, the spine remains elevated (> 3 cm) during abdominal pressure in diseases causing right ventricular dilatation with a poorly compliant right ventricle or in cases of obstruction to filling of the right ventricle by tricuspid narrowing or a right atrial tumour.

Normally, during inspiration, the venous pulse decreases slightly as the decrease in intrathoracic pressure draws blood from the pericardium into the vena cava. An increase in the venous pulse on inspiration (Kussmaul's sign) typically occurs in chronic constrictive pericarditis, right ventricular myocardial infarction and obstructive pulmonary disease (COPD), and also sometimes in heart failure and tricuspid narrowing.

The jugular venous pulse (see figure Normal jugular venous pulse) can usually be seen on clinical examination, but is best appreciated on screen during central venous pressure monitoring.

A waves are increased in pulmonary hypertension and tricuspid valve stenosis. Increased a-waves (canon waves) are seen in atrioventricular dissociation, when the atrium contracts over a closed tricuspid valve. A waves disappear in atrial fibrillation and are accentuated when right ventricular compliance is poor (e.g. pulmonary hypertension or pulmonary stenosis). V waves are very common in tricuspid insufficiency. The x descent is rapid in cardiac tamponade. When the compliance of the right ventricle is low, the y descent is very abrupt, because the abundant venous column entering the right ventricle when the tricuspid valve opens is abruptly stopped by a rigid right ventricular wall (in restrictive cardiomyopathy) or by the pericardium (in constrictive pericarditis).

7.4.4 Inspection and palpation of the chest

The thoracic cavity and all visible cardiac pulses are inspected. The precordial region is palpated for pulses (determining the apical impulse and therefore the position of the cardiac apex) and for murmurs.

a) Inspection

Thoracic deformities can occur in many disorders.

Thoracic deformities, such as shield thorax and carina thorax (pectus carinatum, a preeminence of the sternum similar to that of a bucket), may be associated with Marfan syndrome (which may be accompanied by aortic root or mitral valve disease) or Noonan syndrome (which may be accompanied by pulmonary stenosis, atrial septal defects or hypertrophic cardiomyopathy). Rarely, a tumour in the upper chest is indicative of aortic aneurysm due to syphilis.

Pectus excavatum (funnel chest, sternal depression) with a reduced anteroposterior diameter of the thorax and an abnormally straight thoracic spine, may be associated with hereditary disorders including congenital heart anomalies (e.g. Turner syndrome, Noonan syndrome) and sometimes Marfan syndrome.

b) Palpation

The patient lies down at an angle of between 30 and 45 degrees. Approaching the patient from the right side, the doctor systematically palpates the precordial region.

In healthy subjects, apical shock should be palpable between the 4th and 5th intercostal space just medial to the medio-clavicular line over an area < 2 to 3 cm in diameter.

A mediothoracic elevation, palpable below the sternum and to its left, is suggestive of severe right ventricular hypertrophy. Occasionally, in congenital diseases causing severe enlargement of the right ventricle, the precordial region bulges asymmetrically to the left of the sternum.

Sustained pushing a Гapex (easily differentiated from the less localized and more diffuse lifting of right ventricular hypertrophy) suggests left ventricular hypertrophy.

Abnormal focal systolic pulses can sometimes be seen in dyskinetic ventricular aneurysms. An abnormal diffuse systolic impulse elevates the precordial region in severe mitral insufficiency. Ascent occurs because the left atrium dilates, causing the heart to move anteriorly. The dilated left ventricle or hypertrophy results in a diffuse apical shock and deviates down and to the left (e.g. in mitral insufficiency).

Fremitus is a palpable sensation that occurs with particularly intense murmurs. Their location suggests the cause (see table Location of murmurs and associated disorders).

Palpation of a strong pulse in the 2nd intercostal space to the left of the sternum may be due to exaggerated closure of the pulmonary valve in pulmonary arterial hypertension. A similar early systolic pulse at the cardiac apex may be due to closure of a stenotic mitral valve; opening of the stenotic valve can sometimes be felt at the start of diastole. On auscultation, these findings correspond to an increase in the first heart sound and to the opening of the mitral stenosis.

7.4.5 Examination of the lungs

The lungs are examined for signs of pleural effusion and pulmonary oedema, which can occur with heart diseases such as heart failure. Lung examination includes percussion, palpation and auscultation.

Percussion is the first physical manoeuvre used to detect the presence and level of a pleural effusion. The discovery of areas of dullness on percussion indicates the presence of underlying fluid or, less frequently, condensation.

Palpation includes looking for palpable murmur (vibrations of the chest wall felt when the patient speaks); murmur is reduced in cases of pleural effusion and pneumothorax and increased in cases of pulmonary condensation (e.g. lobar pneumonia).

Auscultation of the lungs is an important part of the examination of patients with suspected heart disease.

The character and intensity of the vesicular murmur are useful in differentiating between pulmonary and cardiac disorders. Adventitial sounds are abnormal noises such as crepitus, rales, wheezing and stridor. Crackles (previously known as rales) and wheezing are abnormal lung sounds that can be observed in heart failure, as well as in non-cardiac disease.

- **Crepitants** are discontinuous adventitious noises. Fine crepitants are short, high-pitched sounds; coarser crepitants are longer-lasting, lower-pitched sounds. Crackles have been compared to the sound of crumpled plastic and can be simulated by rubbing hair between 2 fingers close to the ear. They occur most frequently in atelectasis, alveolar filling (e.g. in pulmonary oedema in heart failure), and interstitial lung disease (e.g. pulmonary fibrosis), and reflect the opening of collapsed alveoli.

• **Wheezing** is a musical, whistling sound that is more pronounced on exhalation than on inspiration. Wheezing is a clinical sign or symptom and is usually associated with dyspnoea. Wheezing is most commonly due to asthma, but can also be observed in cardiac diseases such as heart failure.

7.4.6 Abdominal and limb examination

The extremities and abdomen are examined for signs of fluid overload, which can occur in heart failure as well as in non-cardiac disorders (e.g. renal, hepatic, lymphatic).

a) Abdomen

In the abdomen, significant fluid overload manifests itself as ascites. Marked ascites causes visible distension of the abdomen, which is tense and painless on palpation, with a dullness on abdominal percussion and a fluid wave. The liver may be distended and slightly tender to palpation, and associated with hepatojugular reflux.

b) Members

In the limbs (mainly the legs), excess fluid manifests itself as edema, which is a swelling of the soft tissues due to increased interstitial fluid. Oedema may be visible on inspection, but modest oedema in very obese or very muscular individuals may be difficult to recognise visually. The limbs are therefore palpated to look for the presence and degree of scoop sign (a visible and palpable depression caused by pressure from the examiner's finger, which displaces interstitial fluid). The area of oedema is examined to assess extension, symmetry (i.e. comparing the two limbs), warmth, erythema and tenderness. In cases of significant fluid overload, the oedema may also be present in the sacrum and/or genitals.

Pain and/or erythema, particularly if unilateral, suggest an inflammatory cause (e.g. cellulitis or thrombophlebitis). Non-cavity oedema is more suggestive of vascular or lymphatic obstruction than fluid overload.

7.4.7 Bedside ultrasound

Bedside ultrasound complements the clinical examination using small, inexpensive, battery-operated ultrasound scanners. Both colour and two-dimensional Doppler techniques can be used, and it has been shown that a brief, focused ultrasound examination can improve the detection of a variety of cardiac abnormalities and confirm the findings of the clinical examination, or sometimes establish a diagnosis in the absence of clinical signs. Common uses include the identification of (1, 2)

• Left ventricular systolic dysfunction (with global or regional wall motion abnormality)
• Left ventricular wall motion abnormality (with reduced or normal systemic function)
• High left heart filling pressures (increased left atrium)
• Structure and function of the valve
• Pulmonary edema (vertical B lines in the lung fields)
• Pleural effusion
• Systemic venous congestion (dilated inferior vena cava)
• Pericardial effusions and tamponade

Adequate training in the performance of brief ultrasound examinations is essential to ensure high image quality and accurate interpretation (2). It is important to note that bedside Γechography should be used to enhance rather than replace the clinical examination.

Chapter 8
Diagnosis of respiratory distress

The diagnosis of ARF is based exclusively on clinical criteria, with gasometric abnormalities required for the diagnosis of acute respiratory failure and for etiological orientation.

8.1 Dyspnea

Dyspnoea is an unpleasant and annoying sensation of breathing. It is experienced and described differently by patients depending on the cause.

8.1.1 Pathophysiology of dyspnea

Although dyspnoea is a relatively common problem, the pathophysiology of the uncomfortable sensation of breathing is poorly understood. Unlike other types of nociceptive stimuli, there are no receptors specialised in dyspnea, although MRI studies have identified some specific regions of the mesencephalon that can mediate the perception of dyspnea.

The experience of dyspnoea is probably the result of a complex interaction between chemoreceptor stimulation, mechanical abnormalities in breathing and the perception of these abnormalities by the central nervous system. Some authors have described the imbalance between neurological stimulation and mechanical changes in the lungs and chest wall as neuromechanical decoupling.

8.1.2 Etiology of dyspnea

Dyspnea has many pulmonary, cardiac and other causes, which vary in severity from the onset.

The most frequent causes are :

- Asthma
- Chronic obstructive pulmonary disease (COPD)
- Heart failure
- Myocardial ischemia Physical deconditioning
- Pneumonia

The most frequent cause of dyspnea in chronic pulmonary or cardiac disorders is

- The worsening of their illness

However, these patients may also develop another disease (e.g. a patient with long-standing asthma may have a myocardial infarction, a patient with chronic heart failure may develop pneumonia).

8.1.3 Dyspnea assessment

a) Anamnese

The history of the current illness should look for temporal patterns of onset (e.g. sudden, insidious), and triggering or exacerbating factors (e.g. exposure to allergens, cold, exertion, lying down). Severity can be determined by assessing the level of activity required to cause dyspnoea (e.g. only dyspnoea while climbing stairs is more severe than dyspnoea at rest). The doctor must assess the evolution of the dyspnea in relation to the patient's usual state.

The systems review should look for symptoms of possible causes, including chest pain or a feeling of constriction in the chest (pulmonary embolism, myocardial ischaemia, pneumonia); sudden oedema, orthopnea and paroxysmal nocturnal dyspnoea (heart failure);

fever, chills, cough and sputum (pneumonia); black, tarry stools or heavy menstrual periods (occult bleeding which may be the cause of anaemia); or weight loss and night sweats (cancer or chronic lung infection).

The search for medical antecedents should focus on conditions known to cause dyspnoea, including asthma, COPD and heart disease, as well as the risk factors for the various etiologies:

• A history of smoking, for cancer, COPD, certain interstitial lung diseases and heart disease

• A family history of high blood pressure and high cholesterol levels for coronary artery disease

• Recent immobilisation or surgery, recent long-distance travel, cancer or risk factors for cancer or signs of occult cancer, or a family history of bleeding disorders, pregnancy, taking oral contraceptives, calf pain, leg swelling, and known deep vein thrombosis, for pulmonary embolism.

Occupational exposures (e.g. gas, tobacco, asbestos) should be investigated.

b) Clinical examination

Vital signs are investigated, including fever, tachycardia and tachypnea.

The examination focuses on the cardiopulmonary system.

A complete pulmonary examination is carried out, including assessment of air exchanges, symmetry of the vesicular murmur and the presence of crepitants, ronchi, stridor and wheezing. Signs of condensation (e.g. egophonia, dullness on percussion) should be sought. The cervical, supra-clavicular and inguinal regions should be inspected and palpated for adenopathy.

The jugular veins should be examined for distension, and the pressure areas and limbs should be palpated for buccal oedema (both signs of heart failure).

Heart sounds should be checked for additional heart sounds, muffled heart sounds or a heart murmur. The search for a paradoxical pulse (a drop of >12 mmHg in systolic blood pressure during inspiration) can be carried out by inflating a cuff to 20 mmHg above systolic pressure, which is then slowly deflated until the first Korotkoff sound appears, during exhalation only. As the cuff is deflated, the time at which the first Korotkoff sound becomes audible during inspiration and expiration is recorded. If the difference between the first and second measurement is >12 mmHg, a paradoxical pulse is present.

The conjunctiva should be examined for pallor.

c) Warning signs

The following signs should raise a red flag:

• Resting dyspnoea during examination

• Decreased level of consciousness, agitation or confusion

• Recruitment of accessory respiratory muscles and poor aerial excursion

• Chest pain

• Crepitus

• Weight loss

• Night sweats

• Palpitations

d) Interpreting the signs

The history and clinical examination often suggest a cause and guide further investigations.

Several signs are important:

- Wheezing suggests asthma or COPD.
- Stridor indicates extra-thoracic airway obstruction (e.g. foreign body, epiglottitis, vocal cord dysfunction).
- Crepitants suggest left heart failure, interstitial lung disease or, if accompanied by signs of condensation, pneumonia.

However, the symptomatology of life-threatening conditions such as myocardial ischaemia and pulmonary embolism may be non-specific. Furthermore, the importance of the symptoms is not always proportional to the severity of the cause (e.g. pulmonary embolism in a healthy person may cause only moderate dyspnoea). Great caution is therefore required when dealing with these frequent disorders. It is often appropriate to rule out these disorders before attributing dyspnoea to a less serious etiology.

A clinical prediction system can be used to estimate the risk of pulmonary embolism. It should be noted that normal oxygen saturation does not rule out pulmonary embolism.

Hyperventilation syndrome is a diagnosis of exclusion. Since hypoxia can cause tachypnea and agitation, it would be unwise to assume that any anxious young person with rapid breathing has a simple hyperventilation syndrome.

8.1.4 Ladders

Dyspnea scales provide a direct or indirect measure of dyspnea and/or its impact on daily activity.

a) Medical Research Council (MRC) scale

This scale, which is used extensively in the monitoring of respiratory diseases, is based on difficulties in walking or climbing stairs and defines 4 stages of dyspnea:

- **stage 0:** dyspnea for sustained effort (2 storey ascent)
- **stage 1:** dyspnea when walking fast or on slopes
- **stage 2:** dyspnea when walking on level ground following a person of the same age
- **stage 3:** dyspnoea requiring you to stop and catch your breath after a few minutes or a hundred metres on flat ground
- **stage 4:** dyspnea at the slightest effort

b) Visual Analogue Scale VAS

This is the simplest scale. The patient assesses his breathlessness by moving the cursor to the desired level on a small scale, one end of which indicates "no breathlessness at all" and the other "maximum breathlessness". The doctor assesses shortness of breath by reading the back of the slide.

Over the last ten years or so, multidimensional scales have been developed to give a more global assessment of dyspnea (sensory as well as affective dimensions).

8.2 Signs of hypoxemia

Clinically, hypoxemia may be manifested by cyanosis, predominantly in the extremities, or even consciousness disorders leading to coma and cardiorespiratory arrest.

8.2.1 Definition

Hypoxemia is a reduction in the amount of oxygen in the blood. Breathing allows oxygen to pass from the lung to the blood through the alveolar capillary membrane, which is the exchange zone between the pulmonary alveolus and the pulmonary capillaries where the blood circulates, enriching it with oxygen (a bit long and a lot of repetition, but the idea is to explain the path of oxygen from the lung to the blood)," explains Dr Nicolas Devos, Anaesthesiologist. Get oxygen binds to red blood cells and more specifically to haemoglobin, which is the carrier of this oxygen in the blood to the various tissues in our body. A pulmonary pathology or anemia (reduced hemoglobin) leads to hypoxemia. The result of hypoxemia is a deficit in the supply of oxygen to the tissues, in other words tissue hypoxia. Although the terms hypoxia and hypoxemia are often used interchangeably, they refer to two different situations. "Hypoxemia occurs when the partial pressure of oxygen in the blood (PaO2) is below normal (the normal value is between 80 and 100 mm Hg). Uncorrected hypoxemia leads to hypoxia", says the doctor. For its part, hypoxia is defined as a reduction in oxygen supply at tissue level, which is not measured directly by a laboratory value.

8.2.2 Pathophysiological mechanisms of hypoxemia

Hypoxemia can be explained by two main mechanisms:

- 1. alveolar hypoventilation;
- the shunt phenomenon.

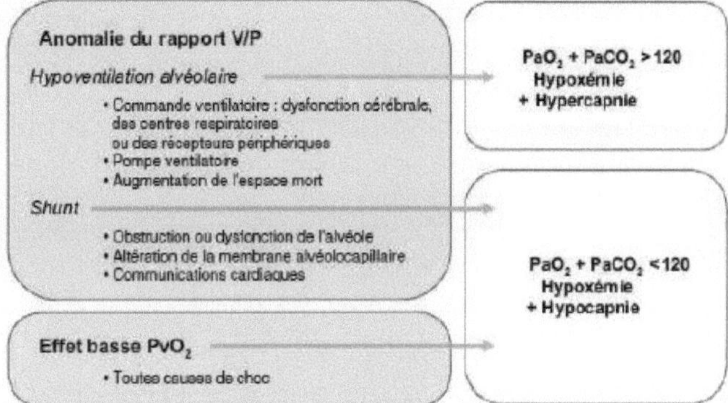

FIGURE 8.1 - Pathophysiological causes of hypoxemia

In intensive care, in the event of a shunt phenomenon, hypoxemia is frequently aggravated during shock due to a low PvO2 effect (outside the programme, see below).

a) Alveolar hypoventilation

Alveolar hypoventilation reflects a reduction in the renewal of Fair at alveolar level throughout the lung. If the alveoli are less ventilated, hypoxemia occurs, associated with hypercapnia - 1'02 does not reach the alveoli, and $CO2$ cannot be eliminated. Blood gas analysis shows hypercapnia proportional to hypoxemia, with the sum of PaO2 + PaCO2 greater than 120 mmHg in ambient air. > The PaO_2 is corrected by oxygen therapy. There are two non-exclusive mechanisms.

1. **Alveolar hypoventilation due to reduced ventilation:**

It corresponds to a drop in minute ventilation (volume inspired and expired in one minute: tidal volume x respiratory frequency), often due to a drop in respiratory frequency, without any change in dead space. Hypoxemia is proportional to the increase in $PaCO2$. For example: coma, psychotropic drug intoxication, etc.

2. **Alveolar hypoventilation due to dead space effect:**

It is secondary to the increase in the ventilation/perfusion ratio (VA/Q > 1) to the benefit of non-perfused ventilated zones. Ventilation of these dead space zones constitutes physiologically useless respiratory work, since in the absence of perfusion, there is no gas exchange. Thus, with the same overall minute ventilation, the healthy alveolar zones are less ventilated, resulting in hypercapnicity and hypoxemia.

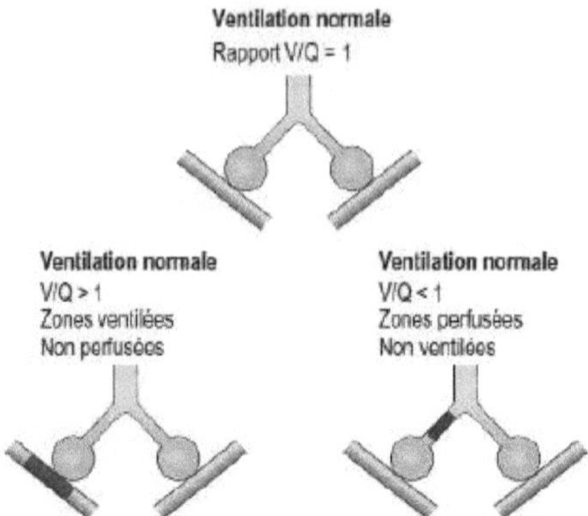

FIGURE 8.2 - Ventilation/perfusion ratios.

Patients with COPD present a situation of alveolar hypoventilation due to an increase in dead space. In the event of decompensation, these patients frequently experience an increase in respiratory frequency with a reduction in tidal volume, which potentially leads to an increase in the ratio of dead space to tidal volume, thereby increasing alveolar hypoventilation.

b) Shunt phenomena

Some of the pulmonary arterial blood 'bypasses' the ventilated zones and is found, still unoxygenated, in the pulmonary veins.

There are two possible, non-exclusive mechanisms:

• The primary cause is the heterogeneity of ventilation/perfusion ratios in the lungs. There are areas that are not ventilated or are poorly ventilated but perfused (VA/Q ratio < 1). Pulmonary mixed venous blood is a mixture of blood oxygenated during hematosis to different degrees (different venous oxygen concentrations) depending on the ventilation/perfusion ratios (different in each pulmonary zone). A change in these ratios can lead to hypoxemia. This shunt phenomenon is by far the most common mechanism that can contribute to hypoxemia. The most frequent causes are alveolar pathologies (alveolar oedema or alteration of the alveolocapillary membrane): car-diogenic or lesional pulmonary oedema (ARDS), infectious pneumopathy or of another origin, bronchial obstruction leading to atelectasis (ventilatory disorder);

• intracardiac shunt: direct passage of blood from the right chambers to the left chambers as a result of a communication between the heart chambers (atrial septal defect, patent foramen ovale).

Hypoxemia leads to compensatory hyperventilation, allowing hypoxemia to be more or less partially corrected. This compensation usually results in hypocapnia, with the sum of PaO_2 + $PaCO_2$ below 120 mmHg in room air.

:■■ I.a PaO_2 is partially corrected by oxygen therapy (no correction in intracardiac shunts).

8.3 Signs of hypercapnia

Hypercapnia, also known as hypercarbia, is the increase in the partial pressure of CO2 (or carbon dioxide) in the blood: it corresponds to an increase in the partial pressure of CO2 (or carbon dioxide) in the blood.

has an increase in the volume of CO2 present in the blood.

Hypercapnicity is diagnosed by measuring blood gases. This is carried out on arterial blood, at the level of an artery, using an arterial puncture. This puncture is performed using a small needle, which draws arterial blood from the radial artery, one of the main arteries in the forearm. Next, the CO2 pressure, i.e. the volume of carbon dioxide present, y will be assessed.

8.3.1 Pathophysiological mechanisms of hypercapnia

Hypercapnicity is secondary to alveolar hypoventilation and is always associated with hypoxemia (which is corrected by oxygen intake). The main mechanisms of alveolar hypoventilation have been described above in the graph "A. Alveolar hypoventilation". Alveolar hypoventilation". The main causes are :

- abnormalities in central ventilatory control :
-    first and foremost, respiratory depressants;
-    cerebral vascular, infectious and traumatic disorders
- neuromuscular dysfunctions and thoracopulmonary anomalies :
— Guillain-Barre syndrome, myasthenia gravis, amyotrophic lateral sclerosis, myopathies, phrenic paralysis...;
— pulmonary restrictive syndromes, pathology of the thoracic cage, obesity;
— COPD;
— respiratory exhaustion.

8.3.2 Causes of hypercapnia

There are three main conditions that can cause hypercapnia. Within these different pathologies, the development or worsening of hypercapnia frequently goes hand in hand with a worsening of the respiratory disease that is the cause.

a)   Chronic obstructive pulmonary disease

The primary cause of hypercapnia is chronic obstructive pulmonary disease. Its major cause is smoking.

b)   Obesity hypoventilation syndrome

The second major cause of hypercapnia, obesity-hypoventilation syndrome, results from the impact of Γ obesity on the respiratory system. Thus, when a large thorax or belly presses on the lungs, they become less efficient, resulting in poorer purification of carbon dioxide and, consequently, a risk of subsequently developing hypercapnia.

c)   Charcot disease

The third and rarer cause of hypercapnia is neuromuscular diseases affecting the respiratory system, such as amyotrophic lateral sclerosis, also known as Charcot's disease.

It will therefore very often be necessary to assist the patient's breathing, using non-invasive ventilation.

8.3.3 Risks of complications from hypercapnia

a)   Running out of steam

The major complication of hypercapnia is the risk of rapid breathlessness during exercise. This is a highly disabling consequence, since at the slightest effort, and during any activity of daily life, the patient will very quickly find himself out of breath, and will therefore have difficulty performing these various tasks.

b)   Other consequences

It also results from hypercapnia, when it becomes chronic:

- **Poor sleep:** people with hypercapnia sleep less well.

- **Sleepiness:** these patients very often feel drowsy throughout the day, mainly due to poor sleep.
- **Headaches:** patients with hypercapnia very often wake up in the morning with headaches.

8.4 Signs of acute respiratory distress (signs of severity)

8.4.1 Respiratory

The following signs of respiratory severity indicate an abnormal increase in the work of breathing (signs of struggle) or neuromuscular failure of the respiratory system (signs of fatigue):

- polypnea > 30/min;
- bradypnea < 15/min, which should make you fear imminent respiratory arrest;
- draught (hollowing of the tissues surrounding the thoracic cage during inspiration), which reflects the use of accessory inspiratory muscles: contraction of the cervical muscles (sterno-cleidomastoid, scalene), inspiratory depression of the intercostal spaces, supra-sternal and supra-clavicular depression, inspiratory shortening of the extrathoracic trachea (Campbell's sign);
- expiratory contraction of the abdominal muscles;
- signs of hypercapnia;
- paradoxical respiration: inspiratory depression of the epigastric cavity with thoracoabdominal asynchronism reflecting diaphragmatic failure;
- difficulty in speaking, ineffective cough: reflecting reduced expiratory flow in the airways.

8.4.2 Cardiovascular

- Paradoxical pulse: inspiratory decrease in arterial pressure of more than 20 mmHg, reflecting variations in intrathoracic pressure due to respiratory effort.
- Signs of acute pulmonary heart disease: tachycardia > 120/minute, hypotension, mottling, skin recolour time > 3 seconds, jugular turgidity, hepatica, hepatojugular reflux.

8.4.3 Neurological disorders
* Agitation, confusion, delirium, hallucination.
* Obnubilation, coma.
* Convulsions.

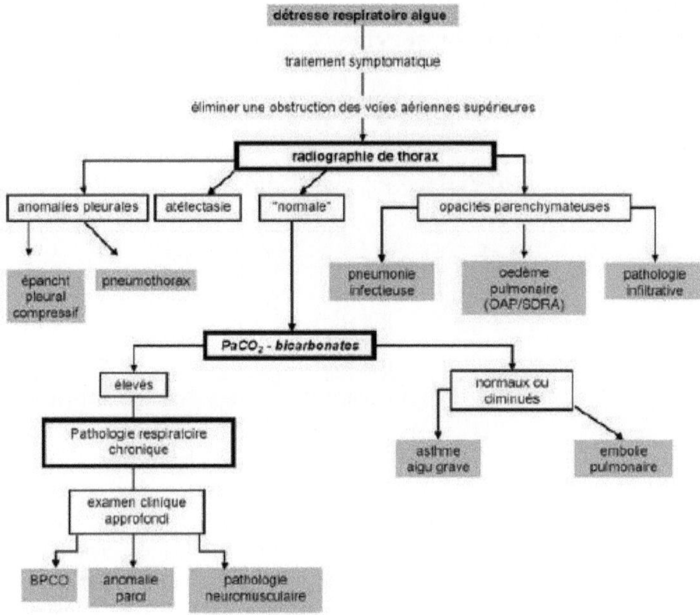

FIGURE 8.3 - Diagnostic algorithm for acute respiratory distress

Chapter 9
Therapeutic management

9.1 Pre-hospital care

9.1.1 Calling the emergency services

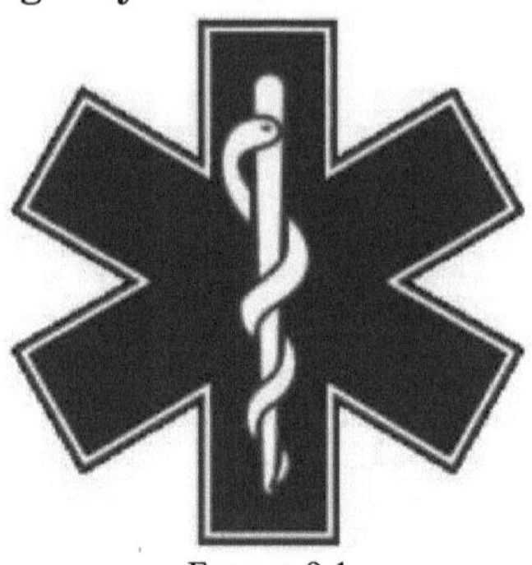

FIGURE 9.1

The emergency medical service (SAMU) is the medical and health regulation centre for emergencies in a health region. It is an emergency service that responds to requests for urgent medical assistance (AMU), i.e. pre-hospital assistance (in the street, at home, in the workplace, etc.) to victims of accidents or sudden illnesses in a critical condition (sickness, illness, or pregnant women). The SAMU regulating doctor manages the urgent care resources, constantly checking their availability and directing patients to the services best suited to their needs.

9.1.2 Clearing the airways

The airways may be accidentally obstructed, obstructing or preventing the passage of Lair. In this case, the Pair passage needs to be freed, "to ensure the permeability of the upper airways", to allow spon- taneous ventilation or artificial ventilation. This is known as airway clearance. This is also known as airway control.

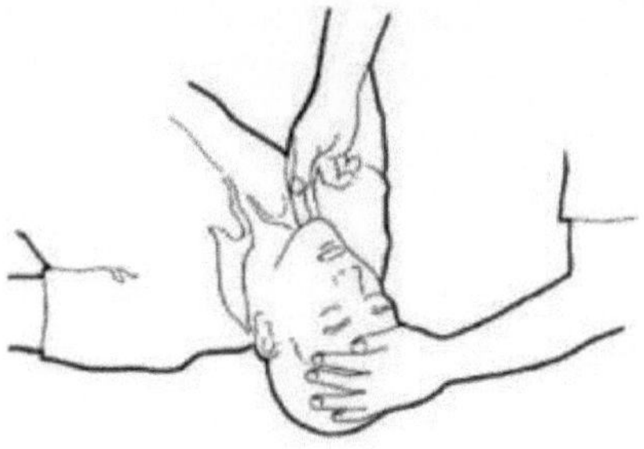

FIGURE 9.2

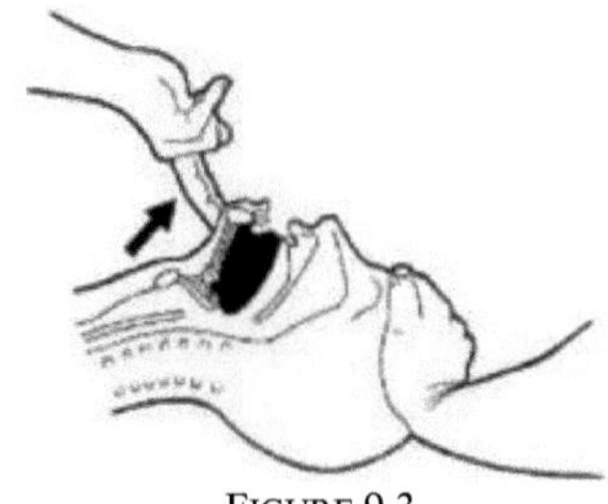

FIGURE 9.3

Clearing the airways is one of the first concerns in a rescue operation; it's the A (airways) of Peter Safar's ΓABC.

a)   Total obstruction

The airways can be obstructed by an object, such as food, or in young children by a marble, a peanut... In a conscious person, total obstruction can be recognised by the following signs:

- the person tries to breathe but cannot;
- no sound comes out of his mouth (no talking, no coughing, no whistling);
- the person's mouth is open and they are holding their hands to their cone.

If the obstruction is total, the object must be expelled by creating excess air pressure in the lungs:

- **on a** conscious **adult and child** (from 1 year old to puberty), by giving 5 hard slaps on the back, with the flat of the hand, between the 2 shoulder blades and, if this fails, by performing the Heimlich method: stand behind the victim, place your arms under the victim's armpits, one hand closed in the shape of a point above the navel, the other hand on top, lift your arms away from the victim's sides and perform a comma movement. Repeat the gesture 5 times in succession.

Repeat the 5 back slaps, then the 5 abdominal compressions until the foreign body is expelled, or until the victim loses consciousness. Once the foreign body has been expelled, always seek medical advice, as this method is very hard on the body.

- **on a conscious infant** (from 0 to 1 year old) we apply 5 slaps on the back (using controlled force), with 5 chest compressions. (identical to cardiac massage).

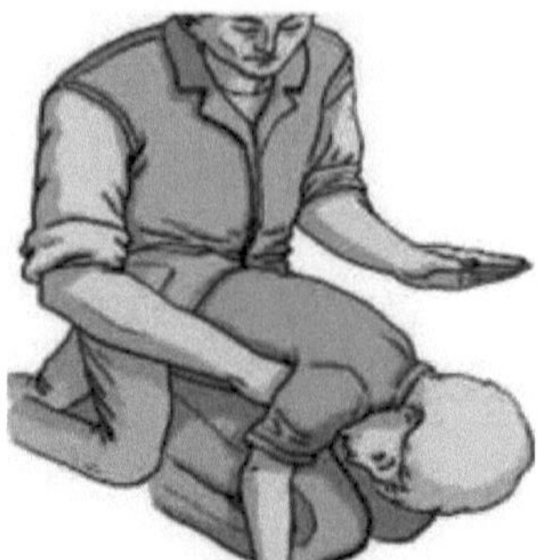

FIGURE 9.4

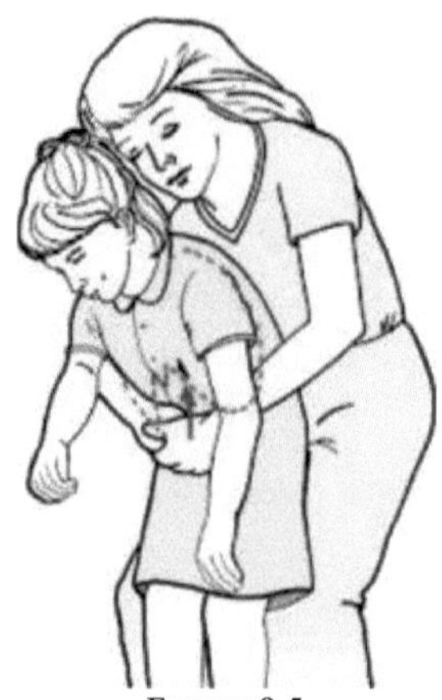

FIGURE 9.5

• From the moment the victim loses consciousness, apply resuscitation manoeuvres (external cardiac massage): 30 compressions - 2 ventilations (even if they are not effective because of obstruction).

b) Partial obstruction

If the airways are only partially obstructed (air passes through, but only with difficulty), the victim's life is not at risk as he or she can still breathe.

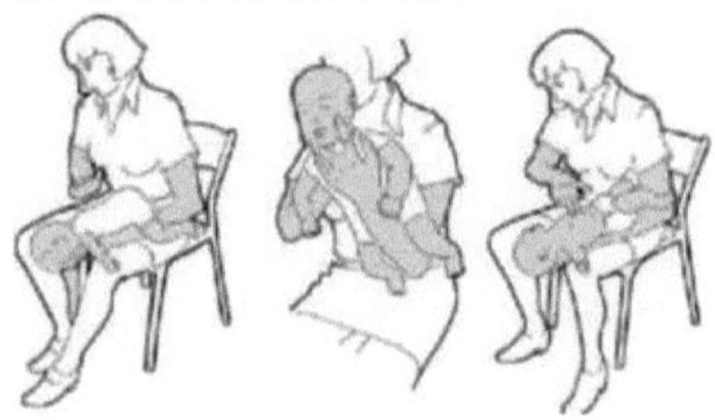

FIGURE 9.6

Do not make any violent gestures to avoid moving the object, and place the victim in a seated

74

or semi-seated position, removing any clothing that could impede ventilation (belt, trouser button, collar, tie).

Medical assistance should be called (112 in the European Union, 15 in France), and the obstruction will be removed by a doctor.

c) Unconscious victim

- General case :

An unconscious victim has no muscle tone, and no reflexes to remove objects blocking the airway (coughing, swallowing). The airways may be obstructed by :

— the tongue, which hangs limply in the mouth;

— 1 the epiglottis, which is normally used to prevent food passing into the lungs, and which remains closed;

— fluids (saliva, blood, nasal mucus);

— food or foreign bodies.

Clearing the airways involves

— unshrink clothing that could restrict breathing (belt, trouser button, collar, tie);

— tilt the head carefully backwards, raising the chin; method: one hand on the forehead, 2 or 3 fingers under the chin

- visually inspect the mouth and remove any foreign bodies (food, chewing gum, loose dentures).

In fact, the muscles controlling the epiglottis (geniohyoid muscles) are attached to the chin. To see for yourself, just ask someone to tilt their head back and swallow their saliva, and you'll see two muscles tense up (this is easier to see in a man because of the Adam's apple). Done, lifting the chin mechanically lifts the epiglottis by pulling on the muscles. This also lifts the tongue. Then, the mouth is opened and any object that might interfere with breathing is removed. First-aid teams equipped with a mucositis aspirator can suck up fluids from the visible part of the mouth.

If the person is breathing, they should be turned onto their side, into the lateral safety position (PLS): this position allows the head to remain tilted without the hands, and allows fluids (saliva, blood, mucus, stomach contents) to drain to the ground. If the person is lying flat on their stomach, they are already in a protected position. If the person is sitting down (in a car, for example), he or she should be made to lie down immediately.

For an unconscious person who is breathing, lying flat on the back with a mucus aspirator close at hand is not currently considered in France to be an effective method of protecting the airways. In fact, the muscles closing the stomach (cardia) have no tone, so the stomach empties into the back of the throat without a sound. When the liquid is seen in the visible part of the airways, it has already penetrated the lungs and caused damage (Mendelson's syndrome). Lying flat is therefore imperative, even for a person with suspected spinal damage (fall from a height, traffic accident). However, this point is approached differently in other countries. The situation is different for medical teams, who have probes that allow them to aspirate into the invisible part of the throat, and who can prevent this risk by intubating.

If the person is not breathing, this head tilt must be maintained while artificial ventilation is performed (mouth-to-mouth, mouth-to-nose...).

- Laryngectomies:

A laryngectomee (or tracheotomee) is a person who breathes through a hole (the stoma) in the neck. This represents around 20,000 people in France.

In the event of obstruction of the airways (in particular, the stoma secretes a large quantity of mucus which can form a plug), unobstruction may require special forceps to remove the obstructing body (Magill forceps, or Laborde forceps with three prongs to separate the edges of the hole).

The hole is located under the vocal cords at the level of the upper tracheal rings, below the aero-digestive crossroads. There is therefore no risk of obstruction of the airways by the tongue or epiglottis, but there is always a risk of invasion by the contents of the stomach and the need to put the patient on the supine position, but the head tilt is of no importance here. At the same time, make sure that nothing blocks the hole, and in particular leave the neck exposed when covering.

In the case of an ostomy, the victim can be left flat on their back, as the airway and digestive tract are separate; however, it is not easy for an untrained person to recognise this situation, so in case of doubt, the victim should be placed on the supine position.

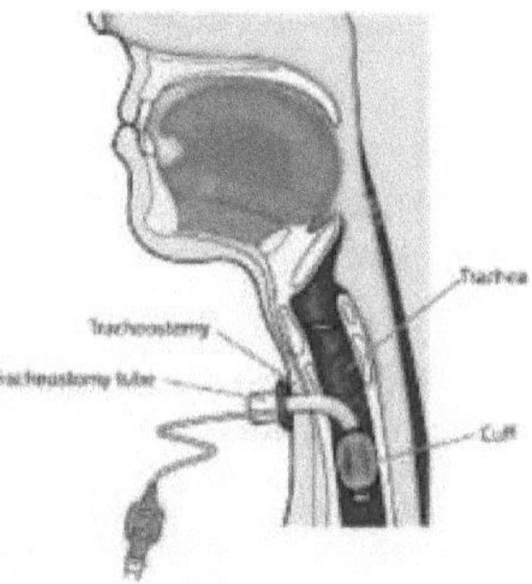

FIGURE 9.7

- Polemic in cases of suspected spinal trauma:

When a spinal trauma is suspected, the aforementioned unsupported manoeuvres present a risk of aggravating the trauma. The situation is debated by experts and there are several doctrines; there is no ideal non-medical solution in this area.

The French doctrine on first and prompt aid considers that

- on the one hand, chin elevation, unlike other head movements, presents little risk of aggravating a trauma if it is carried out carefully;

- on the other hand, inhalation of stomach contents is a definite short-term risk, with almost systematically fatal consequences.

The recommendations are that, if you find an unconscious person breathing flat on their back, you should act in the same way whether or not you suspect cervical trauma, y even for a lone rescuer without a cervical collar.

Some first aiders, when working in a team of more than three people, perform a "pseudo-LSL": they perform a LSL with three first aiders, but stop when the victim is on his side; as the victim is not stable, the three team members stay to hold him in this position; this limits mobilisation and makes it easier to get the victim back on his side when the emergency medical services arrive, but blocks three people.

In other countries, it is considered that the risk of aggravating the trauma is paramount, and the doctrine recommends :

-    if the rescuer is alone and without equipment, to leave the victim in position while waiting for help (unless there is a long delay);

-    in the case of a team of trained first-aiders, to perform mandibular subluxation instead of chin elevation.

Mandibular subluxation involves kneeling behind the victim's head, grasping the lower jaw and raising it; in other words, raising the chin without flexing the neck. This technique is widely used by medical and paramedical teams for intubation. Unlike chin elevation, this method can only be used if the victim is lying down, and if artificial ventilation is required, an additional rescuer is needed to maintain this subluxation (whereas chin elevation can be performed by the rescuer holding the mask). In addition, it is a little more complicated to perform, and may be hampered by the victim's muscle tone (except in the case of cardiorespiratory arrest and deep coma). If this fails, the airways are cleared by conventional chin elevation.

9.1.3 Oxygen therapy

Oxygen therapy is a medical treatment used to supply oxygen to the body via the respiratory tract. Some people suffering from lung disease are unable to absorb enough oxygen from the air and therefore require a supplementary oxygen supply. Oxygen requirements are, moreover, particularly pronounced in the event of physical exertion such as walking or gymnastics.

Oxygen can be administered from several sources:

•   A fixed oxygen concentrator (or extractor). This device concentrates the oxygen contained in ambient air and then allows the patient to breathe it in. It requires an electrical power supply, and is therefore reserved for use in the patient's home.

•   A medical oxygen cylinder. The gas is compressed to a pressure of 200 bars in a special cylinder. This device is rarely used.

•   A cryogenic reservoir or a tank of liquid dioxygen. This device gives patients greater independence, enabling them to travel outside the home. The system consists of a fixed tank containing oxygen in liquid form, and a portable, lightweight tank that the patient can fill themselves. The tank must be filled regularly by the service provider.

•   A portable concentrator (in a rucksack or on wheels) which acts like a fixed concentrator but is powered by a battery.

The aim of oxygen therapy is to increase the amount of oxygen in the body in order to supply vital tissues and organs such as the heart and brain. The therapeutic objective is achieved when SpO2 is greater than 90% and symptoms subside. Patients receiving oxygen therapy generally experience an improvement in cognitive function (memory and concentration), tolerance to exertion, sleep and quality of life.

There are no undesirable effects associated with oxygen intake. However, there are risks associated with hyperbaric oxygen therapy (carried out in a chamber): damage to the inner ear and anxiety attacks.

a)   indications

Oxygen therapy is mainly indicated in cases of respiratory insufficiency. Respiratory failure means that the lungs are unable to provide the body with adequate oxygen. It is manifested by breathlessness, sometimes associated with other symptoms such as intense fatigue, headaches and cyanosis (bluish discolouration of the extremities). Respiratory failure can be acute and sudden in onset, or chronic with a gradual onset.

For the treatment to be effective, it is vital to follow the doctor's prescription in terms of flow rate (number of litres per minute) and duration of administration (number of hours per day).

Two types of oxygen therapy are available: long-term and short-term. Long-term oxygen therapy is indicated for severe COPD.

b) Oxygen therapy in practice

Oxygen therapy is prescribed by a respirologist for an initial period of 3 months after a blood gas has been taken. It is usually carried out in hospital. In the case of chronic disorders, it can be prescribed at home.

Depending on the patient's state of health, oxygen can be delivered via a nasal tube, a mask or by placing the patient in a special chamber.

The provision of oxygen reduces respiratory distress and therefore considerably improves patients' quality of life. It should be noted, however, that the treatment is only effective if oxygen is inhaled for at least 16 hours a day. Ideally, this should be 24 hours a day.

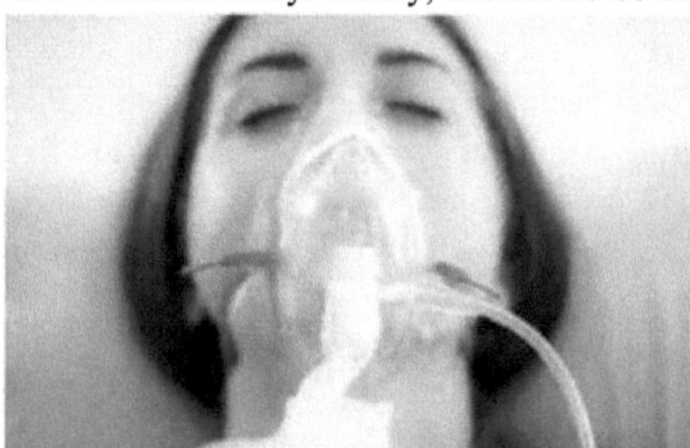

FIGURE 9.8

9.1.4 Placement of a peripheral venous line

a) Indications
- Administration of liquids and IV drugs
- Repeated venous blood sampling

b) Contraindications

1. **Absolute contraindications:**

No

2. **Relative contraindications :**
- Intended use of highly concentrated or irritating IV fluids: use a central venous catheter or intraosseous infusion
- Skin infection or burn at a prospective cannulation site
- Injured or massively cedematous extremities
- Venous thrombosis or phlebitis
- Arteriovenous graft or fistula
- Mastectomy or homolateral lymph node dissection

In the above situations, use another site (e.g. the opposite arm).

c) Complications

Complications are rare and include
- Local infection
- Venous thrombophlebitis

The complications listed above can be reduced by using a sterile technique during insertion and by filling or removing catheters within 72 hours.

Other complications include

* Extravasation of infused fluids into surrounding tissues
* Arterial puncture
* Hematoma or bleeding
* Lesion of the vein
* Nerve damage
* Air embolism
* Catheter embolism

d) Short venous catheter

Short venous catheter placed in a peripheral vein to administer IV treatment.

* Short catheters are flexible polyurethane or polyurethane silicone cannulas inserted into a peripheral vein using a needle mandrel. There are several cannula diameters (gauges), 16G, 18G, 20G, 22G, 24G, 26G and several needle lengths, with or without a safety system.
* The epicranial is a metal needle with wings to grip it and a flexible tube. There are 4 gauges (diameters) of needle to adapt to the vein to be punctured (№ 19, 21, 23, 25) and two lengths of flexible tube.

e) Placement of the peripheral venous catheter

- Choice of site :

Focus on the non-dominant upper limb, hand and forearm, starting with the distal part of the limb, avoiding functional areas such as folds and joints. As far as possible, avoid the lower limbs: painful areas, phlebogenesis, etc.

Focus on the non-dominant upper limb, hand and forearm, starting with the distal part of the limb and avoiding functional areas such as folds and joints.

In adults, insertion of a CVP in the lower limb is not recommended for adult patients and is not indicated for patients with neuropathy. The few exceptions are :

— patient access" constraints in the operating theatre,

— the urgent need for a CVP.

This measure is therefore temporary until other means of vascular access are possible.

- In paediatrics :

In newborns and infants, the most accessible veins are the superficial veins of the hands (pay particular attention to children sucking their thumb), feet and forearms.

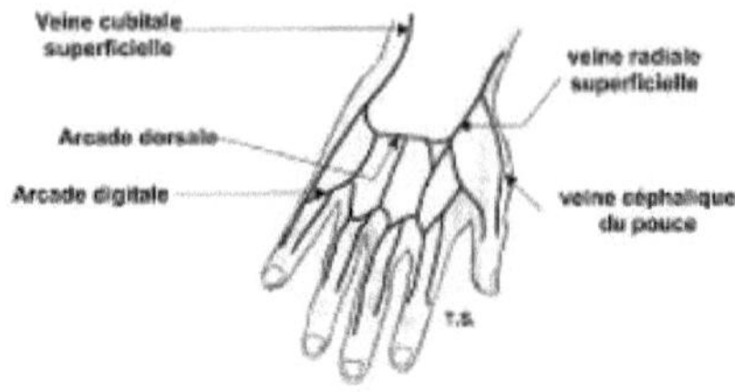

FIGURE 9.9

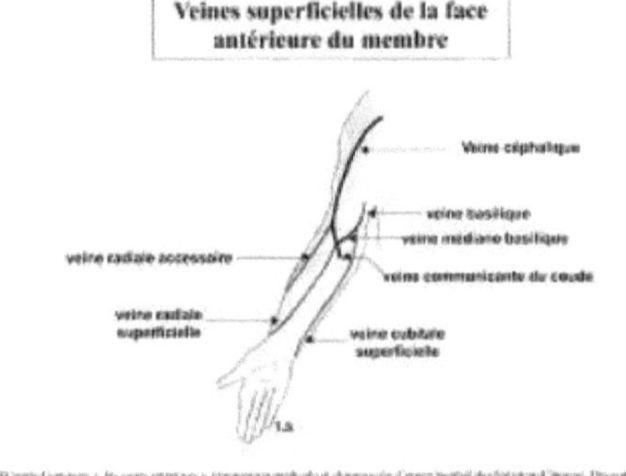

FIGURE 9.10

FIGURE 9.10

If the veins are difficult to feel, use auxiliary means:
- Elevate the limb unless it is oedematous
- Gently tap the chosen puncture site
- Warm the puncture site by soaking the hand in a basin of warm water or with a towel that has been warmed beforehand (do not use a heating pad).
- Do not squeeze the tourniquet too tightly, check for a persistent pulse

9.1.5 Monitoring

The scope (or monitor) is a TV screen that continuously monitors vital parameters such as heart rate, pulse, blood oxygen level (SpO2), blood pressure and temperature. It is connected to the patient by electrodes. In the event of a rhythm disorder, for example, the device triggers a visual and audible alarm.

Scoping a patient means constantly monitoring their vital parameters using a small computer called a "Scope".

Nowadays, these scopes are more sophisticated: smaller and smaller, remote transmission of the display via Wifi, recording of parameters on paper, etc.

The choice of equipment is important, and its technical performance must be tailored to your needs. Prices range from around €1,000 to €3,000.

EMS teams always use battery-powered scopes coupled to a defibrillator to shock the patient in the event of cardiac arrest due to VF or serious rhythm disorders.

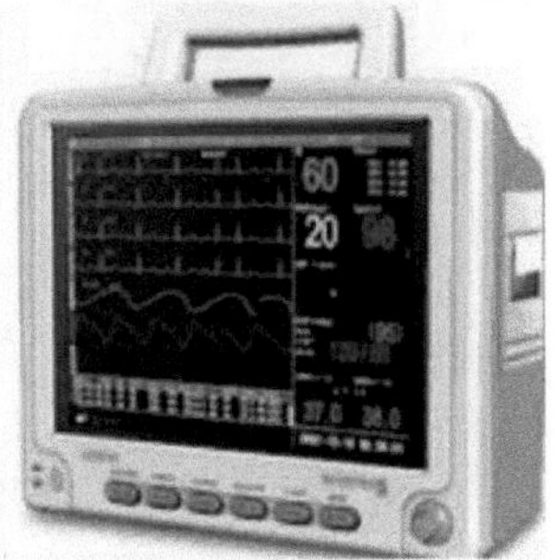

FIGURE 9.11

a) Position of ECG electrodes

Self-adhesive electrodes are preferable because they are more stable and do not restrict the patient's mobility. You can choose between a 3 or 5 electrode system.

1. 3 self-adhesive electrodes
- The red (R) is placed under the right clavicle.
- The yellow (L) is placed under the left clavicle.

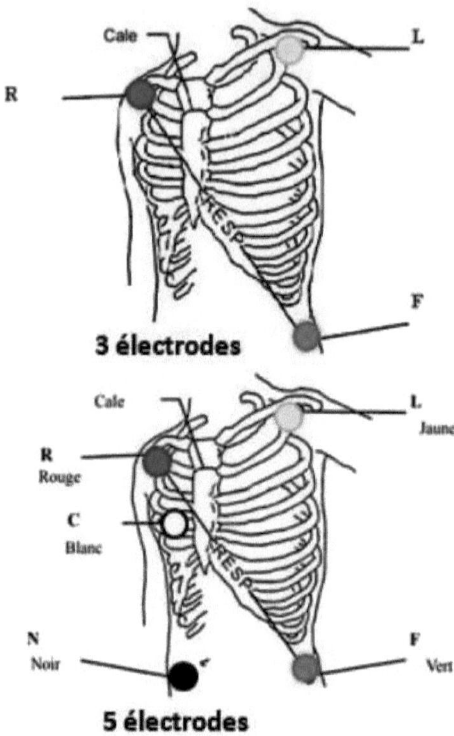

FIGURE 9.12

FIGURE 9.12

- The green electrode (F) is placed under the left costal margin.
2. 5 self-adhesive electrodes
- The red (R) is placed under the right clavicle.
- The yellow (L) is placed under the left clavicle.
- The green electrode (F) is placed under the left costal margin.
- The black electrode (N) is placed under the right costal margin.
- The white electrode (C) is placed on the right chest, in position VI
3. With limb clamps
- Red clip on right wrist
- Yellow clip on left wrist
- Green clip on left ankle
- Black clip on right ankle

You can even use the 12 standard leads to record an ECG if the device options allow.

b) Blood pressure monitoring BP

Use a cuff adapted to the patient's arm (obese, child, etc). Program the device to take automatic blood pressure readings at the desired intervals, for example every 5 or 15 minutes (just long enough not to disturb the patient).

c) Monitoring respiratory rate and SpO2

The pulse oximeter, or saturometer, is a simple, non-invasive instrument for measuring oxygen saturation in haemoglobin. SpO2 stands for pulse saturation in O2. The "p" stands for pulsee.

SpO2 is one of the vital parameters to be assessed for each patient in consultation (consciousness, heart rate, BP, respiratory rate, temperature). It is one of the triage criteria in the emergency department.

The technique was invented in 1942 and has been used since the 1980s by American anaesthetists in operating theatres and recovery rooms. It subsequently became standard practice in medicine.

It is a method of detecting and monitoring hypoxemia in respiratory failure, but it is sometimes imprecise and has its limitations. Some modern devices can also measure capnia (PaCO2), which is very useful in COPD.

1. Oxygen saturation :

In red blood cells, each molecule of haemoglobin (Hb) contains 4 atonies of iron, which enables it to bind a maximum of 4 molecules of oxygen, after which the haemoglobin is described as "100% saturated with oxygen". The saturated red blood cell takes on a bright red colour. Oxygen-poor haemoglobin takes on a violet-blue colour. Oxygen also exists dissolved in the blood in small quantities (1 to 2%).

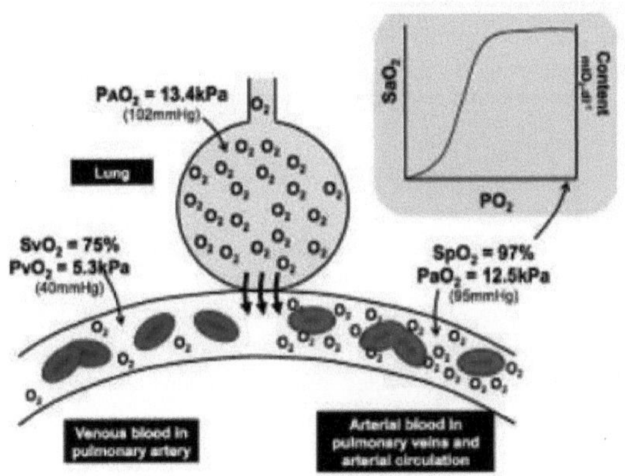

FIGURE 9.13

2. Operating principle :

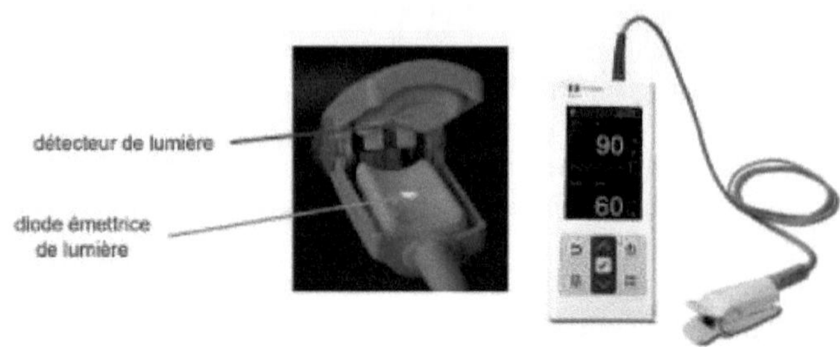

FIGURE 9.14

Pulse oximetry is a non-invasive, transcutaneous technique that measures oxygen saturation of haemoglobin using a sensor positioned on a finger, toe or earlobe. The device uses a spectrophotometric method based on the emission of waves at two different frequencies (red 660 nm and infrared 900 to 940 nm). Light absorption at these wavelengths differs significantly between oxygen-loaded blood and blood containing no oxygen. Oxygenated haemoglobin absorbs more infrared light and allows more red light to pass through. Deoxygenated haemoglobin lets more infrared light through and absorbs more red light.

The sensor consists of a light-emitting diode and on the other side a

receptor for light that has passed through the tissue.

The device displays 3 data points: SpO_2 in %, the pulse rate per minute and the pulse wave curve. The curve becomes irregular in the event of blood hypoperfusion or a poor signal.

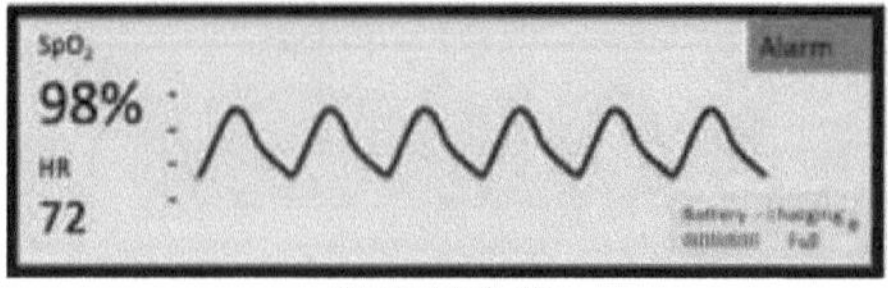

FIGURE 9.15

The pulse oximeter can be incorporated into a patient monitor (scope) that monitors several vital parameters. Portable battery-operated pulse oximeters are also available for use in medical practices, for transport or for home monitoring.

3. **Oximeter indication :**

The oximeter is only a tool for estimating the severity of respiratory failure; it is not a substitute for clinical examination or blood gas monitoring (BGM).

It is indicated in the following situations:

* screening and monitoring of respiratory failure and hy- poxemia in adults and children a Γ with the exception of COPD, for which the major indicator of decompensation is $PaCO_2$ and not SaO_2.
* evaluation of the favourable response to oxygen therapy and/or prescribed thera- peutics.
* monitoring an intubated patient or a patient under general anaesthetic.

SpO_2 <90% is a medical emergency and must be treated with oxygen and appropriate therapies.

4. **Dysfunction factors :**

A number of factors can interfere with the correct operation of a pulse oximeter, including :

* sensor positioning error.

- bright ambient light (such as operating theatre light or sunlight) directly on the probe may affect the reading. Protect the probe from direct light.
- patient movement and shivering can make it difficult to detect the signal.
- pulse volume: the oximeter only detects the pulsatile flow of blood (variation between systole and diastole). When blood pressure is low due to shock or cardiac output is low or the patient has an arrhythmia, the pulse becomes very weak and the oximeter may not be able to detect the signal.
- vasoconstriction reduces blood flow to the peripheries. The oxy-meter may not detect a signal if hypothermic or peripheral vasoconstriction or a tight blood pressure cuff.
- Carbon monoxide (CO) poisoning can give a falsely reassuring saturation. Carbon monoxide binds very well to haemoglobin and displaces oxygen to form a bright red compound called carboxyhemoglobin. Pulse oximetry does not differentiate between O2Hb and COHb because, at the wavelengths chosen, light absorption is very close for both molecules. The pulse oximeter should not be used in this context.
- 1 severe anaemia may distort results due to hemoglobin deficiency.
- Hemoglobin abnormalities: such as drepanocytosis and methemoglobinemia.
- skin pigmentation (dark nail varnish, henna) can alter the SpO2 measurement.

9.1.6 Etiological treatment

if the diagnosis is obvious and treatment is feasible in the pre-hospital setting (diuretics for OAP, bronchodilators for asthma, etc.).

9.2 Hospital treatment

9.2.1 Intensive care unit admission

Continuous monitoring or intensive care depending on the severity and revolution under oxygen therapy.

This is a medical emergency. Respiratory distress requires hospital treatment, with medical transport. Depending on the patient's condition, he or she may be admitted directly to intensive care. The patient should be placed at rest, in a semi-seated position if possible.

9.2.2 Mechanical ventilation

a) NON-INVASIVE VENTILATION (NIV)

NIV is a mechanical aid to breathing using a device (respirator) that delivers pressurised air via a mask applied to the face (mouth + nose or nose only). Non-invasive ventilation (NIV) reduces the workload on the respiratory muscles and improves gas exchange (better oxygenation and lower carbon dioxide levels). Over the long term, NIV can reduce the number of hospital admissions for patients with respiratory insufficiency. NIV should not be confused with CPAP (Continuous Positive Airway Pressure), which is the treatment for sleep apnoea.

1. **Indications:**
- In emergencies (acute respiratory failure, severe COPD decompensation), particularly in patients with COPD, obesity-hypoventilation syndrome or neuromuscular disease. Certain other situations may require NIV in an emergency: certain infections, acute cardiac insufficiency (cardiac oedema of the lung) or post-operatively. In these cases, NIV is used for a few hours or a few days. It can be prescribed continuously for a few hours, then discontinuously thereafter (1h/3h, at night, etc.). Although sometimes a little uncomfortable, NIV is particularly effective in helping patients to breathe. It often avoids the need to intubate the patient (placing a tube down the throat, under general anaesthetic, followed by an

"artificial coma" in intensive care).

• Long-term in fairly infrequent cases. These are patients with advanced respiratory illness (or illness affecting breathing), in which the lung is no longer able to purify carbon dioxide or take in oxygen on its own. In this case, NIV can be performed discontinuously (at night and during the siesta), for long periods, at home.

2. **Contraindications:**

Non-invasive ventilation should not be used in the following cases:

• Absence of spontaneous ventilation, particularly in the event of resuscitation from cardiac arrest

• Unconsciousness (Glasgow score less than 10)

• Administration of hypnotics or sedatives

• Other associated visceral defects

• Upper digestive haemorrhage, vomiting, occlusive syndrome: any case involving a risk of inhalation of digestive fluid

• Hemodynamic instability, right heart failure

• Heart rhythm disorders

• Facial trauma, ENT or maxillofacial surgery (in this case, the mask cannot be watertight or may be painful to keep on)

• Upper airway obstruction

• Ineffective cough

3. **Practical aspects :**

• The most commonly used NIV is positive pressure NIV. By imposing positive pressure on the airways during the inspiratory phase, the ventilator takes over from the respiratory muscles and the diaphragm, thereby reducing O2 consumption by these resting muscles.

• The practical application of NIV, which allows discontinuous ventilation over 24 hours, requires choices to be made concerning both the mask (nasal or facial) and the ventilation modes and their settings.

• The ventilatory modes applicable in flow or pressure are variable: the assist-control mode (ACV), the inspiratory aid (IA) and the BI-PAP are the most commonly used. Spontaneous ventilation (SV) with positive expiratory pressure (PEEP) can also be used.

• NIV is characterised by the existence of air leaks around the mask or through the mouth, which are almost constant. This means that we need to find a compromise ventilation system which, by minimising leaks, allows sufficient alveolar ventilation and provides acceptable comfort for the patient.

4. **Advantages :**

• flexibility of use

• authorises Γ elocution, 1 alimentation, physiological coughing

• simplified mobilisation

• no sedation

• weaning initiated by discontinuous ventilation over 24 hours

5. **Disadvantages:**

• the patient must cooperate

• local intolerance of the mask (irritation of the bridge of the nose, bedsores)

• air leaks which may compromise the effectiveness of ventilation (in the presence of a gastric tube, for example)

• initial workload for the care team

- sometimes use of a chinstrap on the unit for patients ventilated with a nasal mask and who do not keep their mouth closed
- Eye irritation (sign of air leakage)
- Abdominal bloating linked to the passage of some air into the stomach

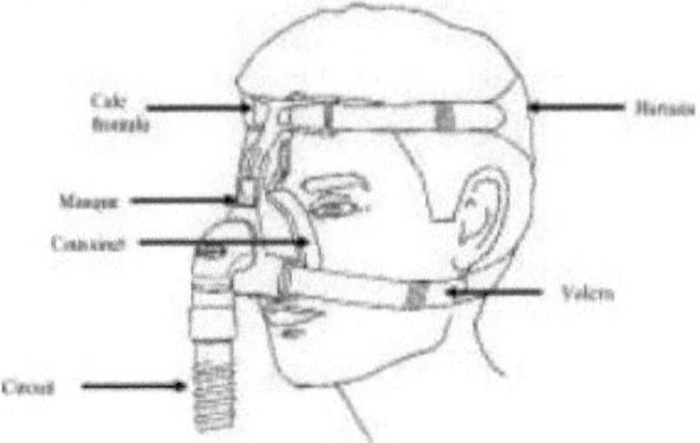

FIGURE 9.16

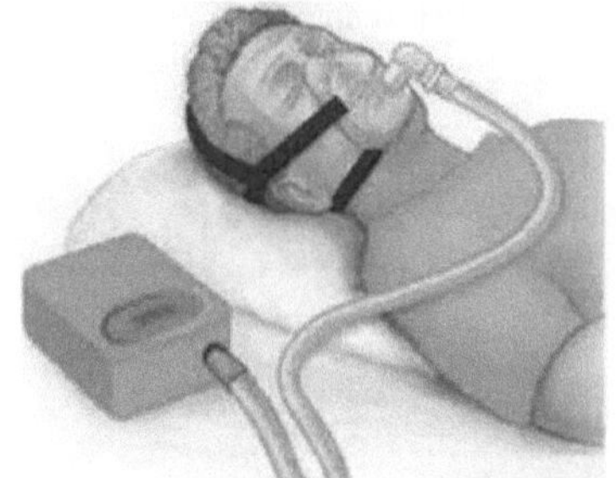

FIGURE 9.17

b) Intubation and invasive ventilation

1. Intubation :

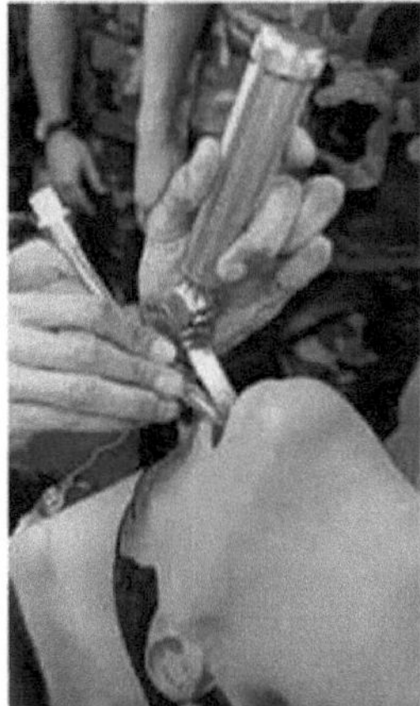

FIGURE 9.18

Intubation is a medical procedure which consists of placing a semi-rigid intubation tube in the trachea to provide artificial ventilation.

87

An intubation is performed with four hands, i.e. two people. One person is at the head of the intubation team and performs the actual intubation. The other person must manage drug injections and assist the operator at the head.

Stages :

- Antiseptic hand washing ;
- Wear protective gloves, mask and goggles;
- Inserting a venous line or ensuring it is working properly;
- Remove all dentures;
- Suction the mouth if necessary;
- Intubate, if necessary after a short pre-oxygenation with the mask.

(a) **Equipment :**

Each intubation requires

- intubation equipment ;
- bronchial suction equipment ;
- easily accessible difficult intubation equipment;
- gastric suction equipment.

(b) **For intubation :**

It must be within easy reach:

- intubation probes of different waffle sizes;
- laryngoscope with set of 2 sterile blades and checked batteries;
- Silcospray® type lubricant or water gel;
- lydocai'ne spray;
- ventilation masks (3 different taffies);
- Guedel cannulas (3 different sizes);
- BAVU mounts and connects to the 02 flowmeter;
- 10 ml syringe;
- fixing strip or specfic system;
- stethoscope;
- non-sterile gloves ;
- protective mask ;
- pressure meter for intubation probe balloon;
- injectable drugs to perform the procedure.

(c) **For bronchial aspiration :**

- single-use sterile suction probes (no 10, 12, 14);
- empty stop;
- collection pocket.

(d) **For gastric aspiration :**

- probes of different sizes;
- collection pocket;
- 50ml syringe with wide tip;
- fixing adhesive or tie according to local protocol;
- cordonnet for work on l'cesophage.

(e) **After intubation:**

- Inflate the balloon using the syringe;
- ventilate using the BAVU ;
- check the symmetry of the vesicular murmur on auscultation;

- check auscultation for the absence of gastric borborygma during ventilation;
- connect the patient to the ventilator;
- attach the probe ;
- check the balloon pressure using the mamometre;
- insert a gastric tube and check its position on auscultation;
- request a contrdle chest x-ray (in intensive care);
- fixing the probe after radiographic control (resuscitation) ;
- record the position of the probe marker in the dental arch;
- Make a note in the file of the type of probe used.

(f) Sellick manoeuvre :

The Sellick manoeuvre is a technique for compressing the cricoid cartilage. During tracheal intubation, it is used to prevent the risk of regurgitation of gastric and oesophageal contents into the pharynx and bronchial and alveolar inhalation during anaesthetic induction, which leads to depression of the airway protection reflexes in a patient with a full stomach.

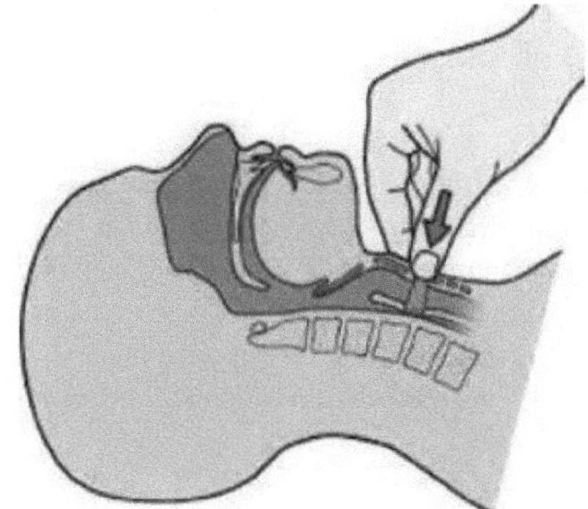

FIGURE 9.19

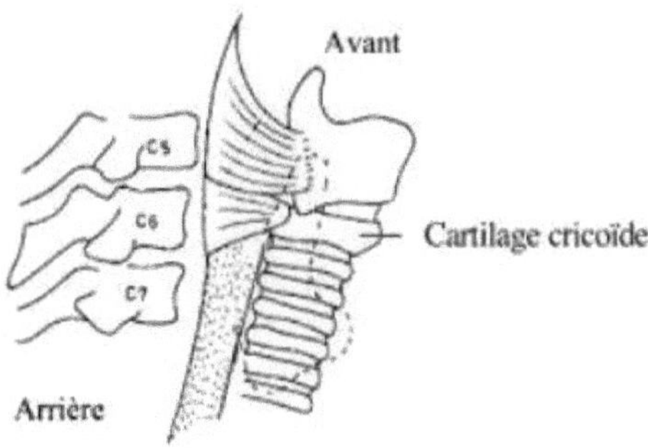

FIGURE 9.20

It consists of pressing firmly on the cricoid cartilage, which then compresses the upper end of the oesophagus, whose walls are flexible, and centres the vertebral body of the underlying

89

cervical vertebra.

i. **Contraindications**
* Active vomiting
* Lesions of the cervical spine
* Laryngeal trauma
* Tracheostomy
* Pharyngeal diverticulum
* Foreign bodies in the airways
* Cervical medullary lesion

ii. **Complications**

Elies are rare but serious.
* Pcesophage rupture
* Rupture of the cricoid cartilage
* Difficulty of intubation if the pressure is too high, which can compromise visualisation of the glottis
* Worsening of pre-existing laryngeal or spinal lesions

2. **Invasive ventilation :**

Mechanical ventilation (MV) in medicine is an artificial form of ventilation (as opposed to spontaneous ventilation) which consists of begging for or assisting spontaneous breathing using an artificial respirator, commonly referred to as a "ventilator" by healthcare professionals. It is most often used in critical care (emergency medicine or resuscitation) and anaesthetic settings, but can also be performed at home on patients with chronic respiratory insufficiency. MV is considered "invasive" if it is performed via an interface that enters the airways through the mouth (endotracheal intubation tube) or through the skin (tracheostomy tube).

There are two main types of mechanical ventilation: positive pressure ventilation, where air (or a mixture of gases) is 'pushed' through the trachea, and negative pressure ventilation, where air is 'sucked' through the lungs. Although the second type was used in the early days of MV and is still used today, albeit rarely, the vast majority of ventilators use positive pressure. There are many different ventilatory modes, the nomenclature and characteristics of which are evolving rapidly as medical technology continues to develop, even tending in recent years towards automated (rather than pre-set) algorithms that continuously adapt to the patient's ventilatory effort.

(a) **Indications:**

Mechanical ventilation is indicated for patients whose spontaneous ventilation is insufficient to keep them alive. It is also used as prophylaxis before an imminent collapse of other physiological functions (before anaesthesia) or in cases where gas exchange becomes ineffective. In theory, given that mechanical ventilation is a temporary organ replacement and does not, strictly speaking, treat a disease, the patient's situation must be reversible to justify its initiation.

The main indications are :
* acute respiratory failure5 (ARDS, chest trauma, etc.);
* respiratory arrest, y including intoxication;
* severe asthma attack ;
* decompensation of chronic respiratory insufficiency (COPD, Pickwick's syndrome, etc.);
* acute respiratory acidosis with partial pressure of carbon dioxide (PCO2) > 50 mmHg

and pH < 7.25;

- paralysis of the diaphragm due to Guillain-Barre syndrome, a medullary lesion, or the effect of anaesthetic and muscle relaxant drugs;
- persistent and aggravating signs of respiratory distress, such as increased work of breathing, tachypnea, etc;
- hypoxemia with partial arterial oxygen pressure (PaO2) < 55 mmHg with inspired oxygen fraction (FiO2) = 1.0;
- hypotension y including sepsis, shock, congestive heart failure, etc;
- neurological diseases such as myasthenia gravis, amyotrophic lateral sclerosis, etc.

(b) **Risks associated with mechanical ventilation :**

- **Baro-trauma**: pneumothorax or alveolar trauma due to excessive intrathoracic pressure;
- **Volu-trauma or volo-trauma:** alveolar trauma linked to excessive intra-alveolar volume, sometimes responsible for secondary scar fibrosis.
- **Intrinsic PEP (PEPi):** caused by incomplete expiration.

It can be caused by an expiratory time that is too short or by increased resistance. In mechanical ventilation, exhalation is passive and the speed at which air leaves the lung depends exclusively on its mechanical characteristics. The consequences of high PEEPi are a reduction in venous return, which can lead to hypotension due to right ventricular failure, and an increased risk of barotrauma due to dynamic hyperinflation. This complication mainly occurs in asthmatic and/or COPD patients.

- **Atrophy of the diaphragm:** controlled ventilation can lead to rapid degradation of the respiratory muscles due to lack of use.

(c) **Artificial respiration:** See artificial respiration section.

9.2.3 Etiological treatment

See chapter on etiological diagnosis

Chapter 10
Treatment of respiratory distress in children

10.1 Respiratory distress in children

Respiratory distress is defined as increased respiratory effort and increased respiratory frequency. This respiratory distress can rapidly deteriorate and lead to disastrous consequences if it is not managed immediately. Tachypnea and the use of accessory respiratory muscles are examples of increased respiratory work. A respiratory rate that is too slow for the age can also be a sign of seriousness (imminent respiratory arrest). The acute respiratory distress syndrome (ARDS) has its own diagnostic criteria.

The management of vital paediatric respiratory distress is not always a task for the paediatrician or paediatric resuscitator: in many hospitals, and in almost all pre-hospital care, it is the "adult" emergency doctor who is responsible for this delicate task: this delicate task falls to the "adult" emergency doctor: he or she initiates first aid and then hands over the rest of the treatment to a paediatric colleague as soon as possible, i.e. a few minutes in the best of cases, or several hours in the least favourable cases:

During this more or less lengthy period of isolation, 1 emergency doctor has to define alone the whole of the therapeutic strategy when faced with a newborn, an infant or a child in vital distress, even though his or her experience in this field varies greatly.

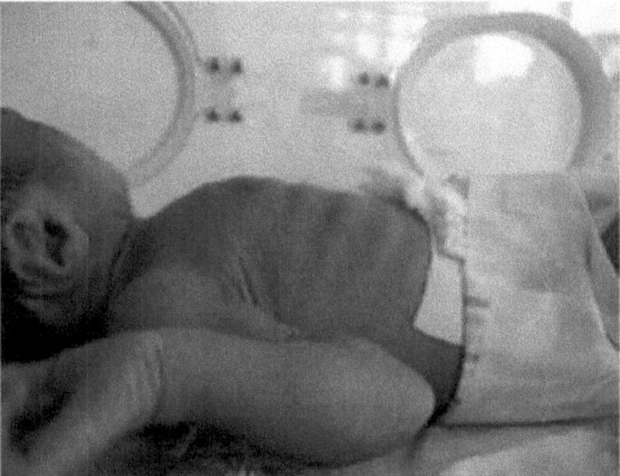

FIGURE 10.1

10.2 Semiological features in children

Physiological changes with age.

The breathing aspect :

- Frequencies :
-     new ne =^ 40 to 50 mts /mn
-     Infant =^ 25 to 30mts/mn
-     From 2 3 years =^ 18 to 20 mts/mn
- Types of breathing :
- New ne :

* Abdominal breathing
* Taken nasally
* Often irregular rhythm
- Infant :
* Breathing gradually becomes thoracoabdominal
* From 6 months can breathe through the mouth
* Regularity of breathing rhythm
- From age 2 :
Breathing identical to that of an adult

10.3 Anatomical features of the respiratory tract in children

The infant's mouth is small, with a relatively large tongue, making it easy to obstruct the airway if consciousness is impaired. The floor of the mouth is easily compressible and the upper airway (LAV) can be obstructed by compression of the soft tissues of the mucnon.

Until the age of around three months, an infant's breathing is mainly nasal. As a result, obstruction of the nose by secretions can lead to an increase in respiratory workload and respiratory insufficiency (RI).

The infant's larynx is situated higher than that of the adult. Its anterior orientation puts it at greater risk of obstruction in the event of soft tissue compression. The U-shaped cpiglottis protrudes into the pharynx at a 45° angle. The vocal cords are short. Under the age of eight, the larynx is hourglass-shaped, with the narrowest part at the level of the cricoid cartilage. Older children have a cylindrical larynx until the stem bronchi divide.

The diameter of the airways is smaller than in adults, and becomes blocked more easily in the event of axlemc.

The lungs are immature at birth, with an air-veolus interface of just 3 m2 compared with the 70 m2 interface in adults. As a result, 1 the child's respiratory deterioration will be more rapid, given that the lung territory that can be covered is smaller.

The main breathing muscle in infants is the diaphragm, due to the inefficiency of the intestinal muscles, which are still too weak at this age. Breathing is more "abdominal". This should not be confused with <<thoraco-abdominal rocking >>, a sign of respiratory distress.

10.4 Diagnosis

Silverman score :

In neonatal paediatrics, the Silverman score is used to diagnose and assess respiratory distress in newborns.

It consists of five items scored from zero to two. Respiratory distress is significant if the score is greater than four and requires intubation.

However, a score of zero does not mean that the child is doing well.

	0	1	2
Thoracoabdominal swing	Synchronous breathing	Abdominal breathing	Paradoxical breathing
Drawing	Absent	Intercostal	Intercostal and suprasternal or substernal
Xyphoid funnel	Absent	Modere	Intense

Nose flapping	Absent	Modere	Intense
Expiratory whine	Absent	Percu with stethoscope	Audible at a distance

FIGURE 10.2 - Silverman score

Respiratory distress in children is often identified by simple clinical inspection. The respiratory rate is increased (> *50c/min*) = tachypnea, or decreased (< *15c/min*) - bradypnea. The signs of struggle are :
• the flapping of the wings of the nose (respiratory dilation of the nostrils);
• draught (visible depression of the soft tissues), of great value because of its intensity (signs of severity) or its topography (supra-sternal, intercostal or sub-sternal), which makes it possible to locate the possible site of an obstruction.

10.5 Additional examinations

Further investigations are guided by the clinical context. Chest X-rays generally confirm the mechanism of the disease envisaged in the case of
Γ clinical examination:
• tachypnea with intense cyanosis (predominantly alveolar pathology), reduced transparency of both lung fields (pulmonary focus or atelectasis);
• obstructive expiratory dyspnoea (bronchiolar pathology): hyperclarity, predominant pulmonary distension.
Measurement of arterial saturation by pulse oximetry (SpO2) is a very important non-invasive parameter: if it is < 94% on air, it is an indication for hospitalisation. Sometimes, blood gases confirm the clinical signs of seve- ritis (hypoxia (PaO2 < 60mmHg) with hypercapnia *(PaCO2 > 60mmHg)*. If a foreign body is suspected, an endoscopic examination by a paediatric ENT doctor is warranted. If the diagnosis is confirmed, appropriate treatment can be administered under general anaesthetic.

10.6 Indices of gravity

• Polypnee (FR > 60 cycles/min)
• Exhalation whine audible at a distance
• Silverman score > 6
• Oxygen requirement > 40% to maintain *SpO2 > 90%.*
• Associated hemodynamic disorders
• Disturbed consciousness, hypotonia, hyporeactivity

10.7 Support

Respiratory distress can rapidly lead to the patient's death. It is therefore essential to quickly perform a Γ ABC and stabilise the patient. ABC must be performed before the history, in-depth physical examination or further investigation.
If one of the ABC criteria is missing, :
1. remove Lobstruction

- Unc aspiration of secretions pcut ctrc ncccssairc
- If there is evidence of a foreign body and the burn is very recent, Heirnlich's method can be used.
- Emergency laryngoscopy can be performed if it is available quickly.
- If each of the following 6 steps is blocked and the air still does not pass, the patient should be intubated. If intubation is impossible (particularly when the obstruction is high), a crycothyrotomy may be performed as a last resort.
2. Ventilate the patient and administer oxygen
- first try the mask for ventilation with a bag
- If saturation does not improve, intubate the patient
3. Cardiac massage

Once the patient's 123 has been stabilised, different approaches can be considered depending on the underlying pathology.

When airway obstruction is inflammatory, nebulised corticosteroids or oral medication may be used to relieve the obstruction. However, in the case of physical obstruction or when the inflammation is too great, intubation may be necessary.

You should always check that patients are able to hydrate, especially newborns. If they are unable to hydrate properly (drink or eat), consider using a restorative solution.

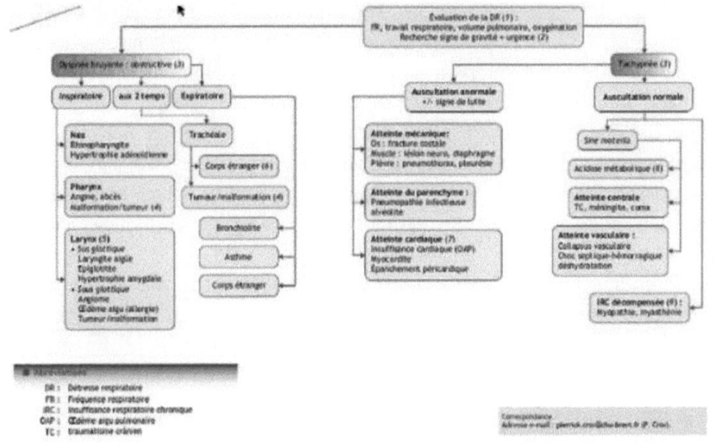

FIGURE 10.3

Chapter 11
Pre-hospital management of covid - 19

11.1 Introduction

Coronavirus disease (COVID-19) is caused by the severe acute respiratory syndrome coronavirus 2 (SARS-CoV-2), also known as COVID-19 virus. After the very first reports of cases of COVID-19 in December 2019, the disease spread rapidly. The WHO declared the epidemic a public health emergency of international concern in January 2020, followed by a pandemic in March 2020.

The COVID-19 virus is zoonotic in origin, meaning that it has been transmitted from animals to humans before spreading between people. An infected person transmits it mainly via droplets of saliva and nasal secretions. In most cases, infection with the virus causes mild to moderate respiratory illness, and the patient recovers without any specific treatment. People who are elderly or have other health problems are at greater risk of developing a severe form of the disease.

11.2 Virus hosts

The ideal hosts for coronaviruses, as warm-blooded flying vertebrates, are bats (for Alphacoronaviruses and Betacoronaviruses) and birds (for Gammacoronaviruses and Deltacoronaviruses). These reservoir species ensure the revolution and dissemination of coronaviruses. In other species, symptoms vary (upper respiratory tract disease in hens, diarrhoea in cows and pigs, digestive tract disease in cats and dogs, etc.).

Sometimes, no symptoms are associated with their presence (e.g. beluga coronavirus).

Humans are naturally home to four types of benign coronavirus, which cause respiratory tract infections such as the common cold, and more rarely affect the gastrointestinal, cardiac and nervous systems.

Coronavirus groups normally have a specific animal host (mammals or birds) but they can sometimes change host as a result of mutation. It is such mutations that have probably led to the emergence of strains causing serious infections in humans (SARS, MERS and Covid-19).

11.3 Tropism

For a long time, coronaviruses were thought to have a solely respiratory or gastrointestinal tropism (resulting in pneumonia and enterocolitis in severe cases), but a growing number of studies are showing a much wider tropism, notably cardiovascular, and neurological as well (since the 1980s, it has been shown that several coronaviruses, including most recently SARS-CoV-2, are clearly also neuroinvasive and neurotropic to such an extent that this diversity of tropisms and symptoms makes coronaviruses (murine in particular, grouped together under the acronym MHV) an animal model for the study of human diseases as varied as multiple sclerosis, viral hepatitis or pneumonia (S. R. Weiss et al. 2011). MHV penetrates the central nervous system (CNS) via the neurons of the olfactory nerve, and can cause acute encephalitis6 or chronic demyelinating disease if it persists (it can also spread to the spinal cord).

11.4 Morphology

Morphologic of a coronavirus. This envelope virus consists of a viral envelope surrounding a helical capsid containing the RNA strand. The genome size of these viruses varies from around 26 to 32 kilobases, among the largest of all RNA viruses.

Coronaviruses share proteins designated by a letter indicating their location: S (protuberances), E (envelope), M (membrane) and N (nucleocapsid). Some, notably those in sub-group A of the Betacoronavirus genus, have a characteristic HE (hemagglutinin esterase) protein. The SARS coronavirus also has a specific binding site on the S protein for the angiotensin 2 converting enzyme, which serves as its entry point into the host cell.

The physical size of the virion is classically given as 120 to 160 nm or of the order of 125 nm. However, SARS-CoV-2, the virus responsible for Covid-19, has more recently been reported to measure approximately 60 to 140 nm, and to be elliptical in shape with numerous variations.

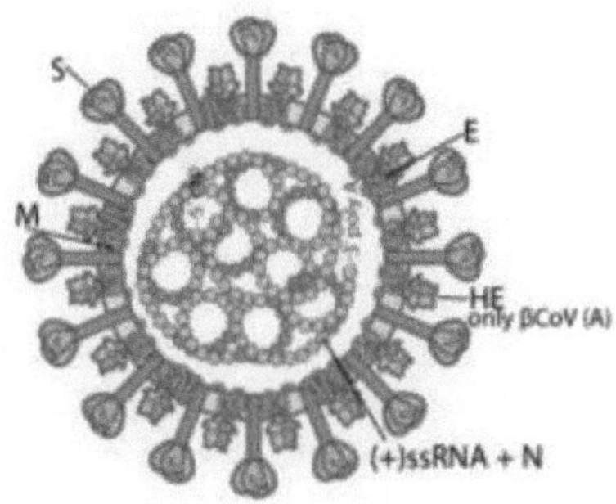

FIGURE 11.1

11.5 Genome

All CoVs have a non-segmented (single-stranded) RNA genome organised in the same way: around two-thirds of the genome contains two large, overlapping "open reading frames" (known as ORFla and ORFlb). These two frames are translated into the "replicase polyproteins" ppla and pplab. "These polyproteins are then processed to generate 16 non-structural proteins, designated nspl 16. The remaining part of the genome contains ORFs for structural proteins, y including spike (S), envelope (E), membrane (M) and nucleoprotein (N). A number of lineage-specific accessory proteins are also encoded by different lines of CoV."

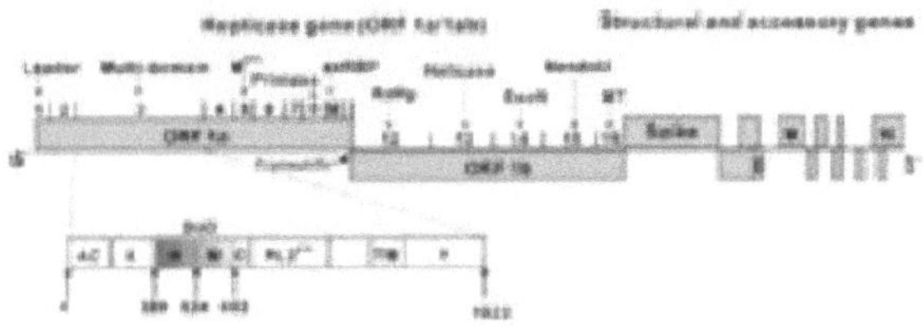

FIGURE 11.2

11.6 Replication

Elijah is made in six successive stages:

1. Thanks to their S protein, coronaviruses bind to cell surface molecules such as metalloproteinases. In addition to the HE (hemagglutinin esterase) protein in their envelope, viruses can also bind to N-acetylneuraminic acid, which acts as a coreceptor (itself initiating

the entry of a pathogen into a host cell). It is not clear whether viruses enter the host cell by fusion of the viral and cellular membranes, or by receptor internalisation. Whatever the mechanism, the RNA strand is inserted into the cell, and the capsid (the shell) is left behind;

2. Coronaviruses have a single positive-stranded RNA genome, present in situ in the cytoplasm. The coronavirus RNA genome has a 5' methylated cap and a 3' polyadenylated tail, allowing the RNA to bind to ribosomes for translation. The cell's ribosomes decode the viral RNA, producing the proteins that y codecs;

3. First, the positive RNA of the virus is transcribed into a protein to form its own RNA polymerase (an RNA-dependent RNA polymerase). Once the gene encoding the replicase has been traced by the host cell ribosome, translation is stopped by a stop codon. This viral replicase only recognises and produces viral RNA, and allows the viral genome to be transcribed into new copies of RNA using the host cell's machinery. Using the positive strand as a template, this enzyme assembles the negative strand;

4. Subsequently, this negative strand itself serves as a model for transcribing small sub-genomic RNAs, which are used to make all the other proteins. This is known as nested transcription. This process is a form of genetic economy, enabling the virus to encode the greatest number of genes in a small number of nucleotides;

the genome of the negative strand is translated by the host cell's ribosome, and a long polyprotein is formed, to which all the viral proteins are attached. Coronaviruses have a non-structural protein - a protease - which is capable of diverging the polyprotein.

This negative strand also plays a role in the replication of new positive-strand RNA genomes. The cytoplasm of the hdte cell is filled with viral proteins and RNA;

5. (a) Protein N helps bind genomic RNA to encapsidate the viral genome in a protective envelope called the capsid30 ; protein M integrates into the membrane of the endoplasmic reticulum, on the capsid side; and proteins HE and S cross the membrane of the endoplasmic reticulum, via the translocation protein, and position themselves on the opposite side;

(b) with the binding between the capsid and the M proteins, the reticulum membrane invaginates and buds. The assembled capsid (the shell), endowed with helical RNA, then finds itself inside the endoplasmic reticulum, having captured for itself the membrane of the latter, which now carries the HE and S proteins on its outside;

6. This viral progeny is then (a) encapsulated and transported by golgi ve- sicles to the cell membrane, (b) and finally externalized (by exocytosis) from the cell.

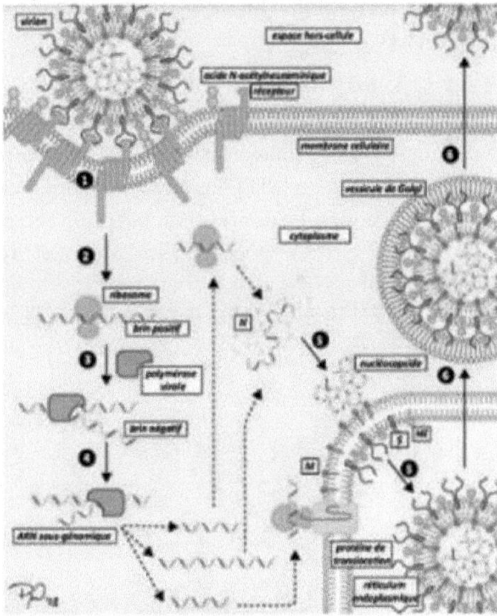

FIGURE 11.3

11.7 symptoms of the disease

Covicl-19 initially causes the classic signs of respiratory infection: fever and cough. The infection may also lead to viral lung damage, resulting in respiratory symptoms (dyspnoea). Other symptoms may accompany or replace these symptoms, but less systematically: muscle pain (myalgia), headache (cephalea), sore throat, nasal congestion, nausea, vomiting, diarrhoea, etc. The sudden onset of a loss of taste (agueusia) or smell (anosmia) in the absence of rhinitis is also one of the most discriminating signs for suspecting Covid-19. Dermatologically, some people develop erythema (redness) or a rash, and more rarely frostbite, particularly on the toes. Studies, supported by the literature, suggest that these may be the result of the hyperinflammation observed in Covid-19.

In practice, the nature and severity of the various symptoms vary according to the individual and their age. Children often have fewer symptoms than adults. Older people, on the other hand, may suddenly present with atypical signs of the disease, such as malaise, repeated falls or confusion. Covid-19 may therefore be suspected if no other cause for these symptoms can be identified.

11.8 Evolution of the disease

In the majority of people infected, the virus causes mild or moderate symptoms that disappear after 5 to 14 days. In others, lung damage, linked both to the virus and to hyperinflammation, may lead to a lack of blood oxygenation and require hospitalisation.

11.9 Additional examinations

Recommended emergency tests: CBC, blood ion count, renal function, liver function tests, D-dimer, LDH, CPK, CRP and blood cultures if fever. Lymphopenia, eosinopenia, elevated LDH and D-dimer levels. PCT is normal on admission for pneumonia, but may be elevated in the most severe cases.

injection-free thoracic CT has become the first-line lung imaging test for a suspected or confirmed diagnosis of COVID-19.

11.10   Signs of CT severity

The main CT sign of severity is the extent of pa- renchymatous abnormalities on the initial CT scan. Numerous studies report a correlation between Γ extension of lesions and clinical severity. The Society of Thoracic Imaging (SIT) therefore recommends grading parenchymal involvement according to a 5-stage visual classification, based on the percentage of lesioned lung: absent or minimal at- taint (< 10%), moderate (10-25%), extensive (25-50%), severe (50-75%) or critical(> 75%).

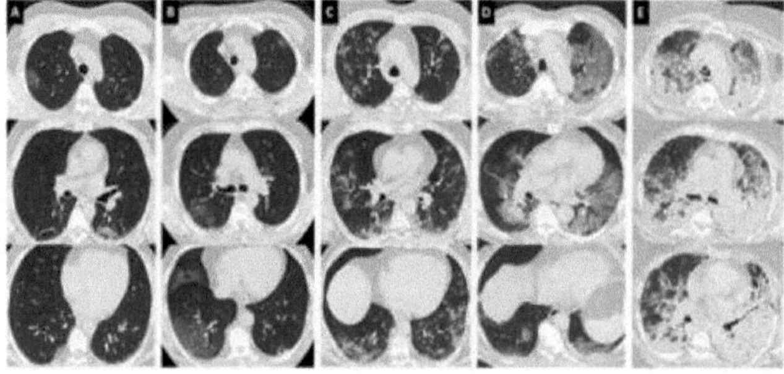

FIGURE 11.4

In addition to lesional extension, parenchymal density is also a marker of severity, with parenchymal condensations appearing more extensive than depoliated glass in the most severe patients. Pleural effusion and early architectural distortion with traction bronchiectasis would also be markers of severity. A Chinese series not yet published suggests that initial involvement of the upper lobes could be a pejorative prognostic marker.

Different degrees of involvement in COVID-19 pneumonia. Lung involvement, assessed visually as the ratio of pathological to healthy lung, can be classified as minimal < 10% (A), moderate 10-25% (B), extensive 25-50 > (C), severe 50-75 > (D) or critical > 75% (E). Diffuse involvement and declining condensation suggest acute respiratory distress syndrome (E).

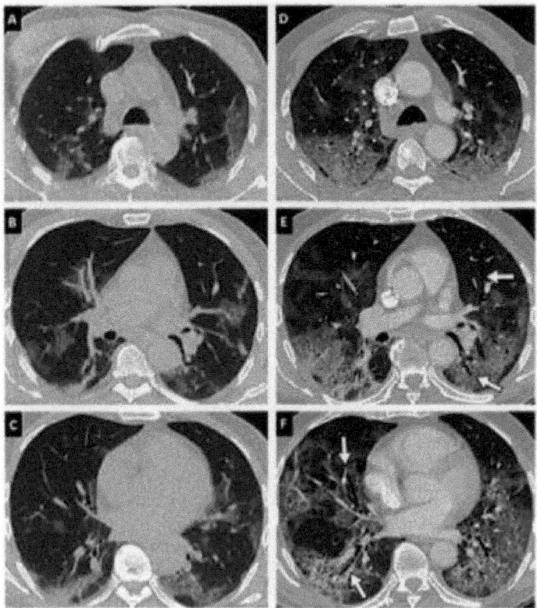

FIGURE 11.5

11.11 Treatment of respiratory distress associated with covid 19

For mild cases (85% of cases), symptomatic treatment with fever and headache medication such as paracetamol will suffice. Anti-inflammatories should be avoided if possible.

In the most severe 15% of cases, pulmonary ventilation is the treatment of choice, because of the paradoxical inflammatory reaction in the lungs.

11.11.1 Oxygen therapy

Only 15% of infected patients required hospitalisation for respiratory signs of seriousness: SpO2 (02 pulse saturation) should be measured with a pulse oximeter as a matter of course at every initial consultation.

of a patient with suspected or proven COVID-19.

Beware of trapping patients with no signs of respiratory distress but who nevertheless have deep hypoxemia, requiring a call to the emergency services and transfer to intensive care before hypoxic cardiac arrest!

In outpatients, there is also a risk of secondary respiratory worsening, especially between days 7 and 12, particularly in patients over 50 and/or with comorbidities. Daily telemedical monitoring of SpO2 by pulse oximetry and respiratory rate (RR) should be performed in these at-risk patients.

Initially, or during outpatient follow-up, any (correctly measured) SpO2 value below "92-94%" at Fair ambiant, especially if the RF is > *22/min,* requires the patient to be transferred to emergency with oxygen therapy, with the aim of achieving SpO2 above 96%.

11.11.2 Antibiotic therapy

Antibiotics are common, inexpensive drugs used to treat bacterial infections. However, recent laboratory studies have shown that certain antibiotics slow down the reproduction of certain viruses, including SARS-CoV-2, the virus responsible for COVID-19. In laboratory tests, one antibiotic, azithromycin, reduced viral activity and inflammation, and was therefore studied as a potential treatment for COVID-19. Solid evidence is needed before antibiotics can be used in COVID-19, as overuse or misuse of antibiotics can lead to 'antimicrobial resistance', i.e. a change in the organisms responsible for infection, so that antibiotics cease to be effective.

Chloroquine, an antimalarial drug, and its derivative hydroxychloroquine, used in certain autoimmune diseases, have shown activity on cells infected with the SARS-CoV-2 coronavirus in vitro. It is also important to remember that the use of these drugs, especially in combination with azithromycin, carries the risk of serious adverse effects, particularly cardiac.

11.11.3 Corticotherapy

Given the absence of any effective antiviral treatment at this stage of pulmonary lesion severity, the "step-by-step" physiopathological understanding of COVID-19 has enabled "innovative" medicinal therapeutic approaches in a viral infection.

First of all, the inflammatory state of these patients, which is sometimes major, and the increased risk of thrombosis and pulmonary embolism, has led to the introduction of double-dose preventive anticoagulation for all intensive care patients, unless there are contraindications.

Above all, the "saga" of corticoids (with anti-inflammatory, anti-fibrosing and vasoconstrictive activity) is instructive because of the knowledge acquired during the first wave of COVID-19, which led us to revise our "certainties" about their use in this new viral context.

The prognostic effects of corticosteroids vary according to the type and severity of pulmonary infection: they are beneficial in pneumocystis associated with HIV infection, are not demonstrated in community-acquired pneumonia, and are deleterious in pneumonia caused by other coronaviruses (MERS-Co-V, SARS-CoV-1) or influenza viruses.

A meta-analysis of numerous randomised, controlled studies evaluating the benefit of corticosteroids during ARDS - from all causes - showed a reduction in ventilation time and mortality compared with placebo.

In the course of COVID-19, preliminary retrospective clinical studies of small numbers have produced conflicting results in terms of mortality. The current recommendations for the use of corticoids in COVID-19 are based on the RECOVERY trial, the only randomised, open-label study involving more than 6,400 patients, which showed a reduction in mortality in all patients receiving oxygen therapy, ranging from nasal ГO2 to mechanical ventilation: administration of dexamethasone 6 mg/d IV or per os for 10 days, as first-line treatment, in mechanically ventilated patients AND in those requiring oxygen therapy. On the other hand, it should not be given to patients who do not require oxygen therapy, as this increases mortality. Our experience in intensive care has shown that it is often necessary to repeat these corticosteroid "cures" when there is clear evidence of cortico-dependence.

At present, none of the many other 'anti-inflammatory' treatments has shown any effectiveness worthy of recommendation. Similarly, no antiviral treatment has been shown to be effective. In conclusion, the pathophysiology of pulmonary involvement in COVID-19 has proved to be multifactorial and original. In the space of a few months, numerous studies have overturned the certainties acquired in other respiratory infectious diseases. In addition to ventilatory modalities that are better adapted to this infection, corticosteroids remain, for the time being, the only possible anti-inflammatory intervention in this major pulmonary attack.

Pulmonary oxygenation of these patients in a severe state may require very long ventilations (> 100 days), with final successes reminding us that "Patience is the mother of all virtues".

11.11.4 Anticoagulant treatment

4 levels of thromboembolic risk :

1.   Low risk / non-hospitalized patient with *BMI* < *30kg/m2 with* no additional FDR.

2.   Intermediate risk: *BMI* < *30kg/m2* with or without additional FDR, without the need for OHND or artificial ventilation.

3.   High risk :

•   *BMI* < *30kg/m2* with or without additional FDR, on HDNB or artificial ventilation

•   *BMI* > *30kg/m2* without additional FDR

•   *BMI* > *30kg/m2* with additional FDR, no need for OHND or artificial ventilation

4.   Very high risk:

•   *BMI* > *30kg/m2* with additional FDR, on HDNB or artificial ventilation

•   ECMO (veno-venous or veno-arterial)

•   Iterative or unusual catheter thrombosis

•   Thrombosis of the extra-renal sewage filter

•   Marked inflammatory syndrome and/or hypercoagulability (e.g. h- brinogen > 8g/L or D-dimer > *3g,g/mlor3000ng/ml)*

Indications

1.   In all patients admitted to hospital, it is recommended that oral anticoagulants, VKAs or AODs (risk of instability and drug interactions) are discontinued, and that heparinotherapy is initiated.

2.   In cases where the risk of thrombosis is low, it is proposed not to prescribe prophylaxis.

3.   In the event of intermediate thrombotic risk, it is proposed to prescribe prophylaxis with low molecular weight heparin in the absence of severe renal insufficiency: for example, enoxaparin 4000 IU once/24h or tinzaparin 3500 IU once/2h.

< *In* the presence of renal insufficiency with creatinine clearance < *15ml/min,* tinzaparin 3500 IU once/ 24h may be used as an alternative to calciparin.

5.   In patients treated with standard-dose prophylactic LMWH, it is proposed NOT to monitor anti-Xa activity.

6. If there is a high risk of thrombosis, it is suggested that intermediates dose LMWH prophylaxis be prescribed: enoxaparin 4000 IU /12h SC, or if weight > 150kg, 6000 IU /12h SC,

7. or HNF 200 IU/kg/24 hours if renal insufficiency)

8. In patients treated with a dose of LMWH higher than the standard prophylactic dose, it is suggested that anti-Xa activity be monitored 4 hours after the 3rd injection, particularly in patients with renal insufficiency, to check for overdosage (> IU/mL) with a higher risk of haemorrhage.

9. In all obese patients *(BMI* > 30) with a high or very high thrombotic risk, the following heparin dosages are proposed: With no additional DRF: enoxaparin 4000 IU/12h; and 6000 IU/12h if weight > 150kg. With an additional DRF: LMWH 100 U/kg SC/12h without exceeding 12,000 IU/1211, or UFH 500 IU/kg/24 hours, dosage then adapted to anti-Xa activity.

10. In all patients on unfractionated heparin, the anti-Xa activity should be checked at least every 48 hours and after each change of dose. If the risk of bleeding is controlled, it should be maintained between 0.3 and 0.5 UI/ml for prophylactic treatment (starting dose 200 IU/kg/24h) and between 0.5 and 0.7 U/ml in the case of very high risk (starting dose 500 UI/kg/d).

11. The introduction of ECMO (veno-venous or veno-arterial) immediately exposes the patient to a very high thrombotic risk. It is therefore proposed to prescribe curative anticoagulation with unfractionated heparin from the start of ECMO (irrespective of the ECMO flow rate), with a target antiXa level of between 0.5 and 0.7 IU/mL.

12. In the event of a marked inflammatory syndrome and a rapid and significant increase in D-dimer levels, curative heparinotherapy is recommended, even in the absence of clinical thrombosis, to investigate a thrombo-embolic event, taking into account the risk of haemorrhage. With UFH, it is recommended that platelet counts be monitored at least every 48 hours, and a drop of more than 40% in platelet count between days 4 and 14 of treatment requires a DIC work-up and a search for anti-FP4/heparin antibodies to rule out heparin-induced thrombocytopenia.

13. In the event of multivisceral failure, or consumption coagulopathy with a sudden drop in fibrinogen, platelet count and factor V level, it is suggested that the dosage of heparinotherapy be re-evaluated, as these events are associated with an increased risk of haemorrhage.

14. The proposed duration of pharmacological thromboprophylaxis (intermediary and high risk) is at least 4 weeks after recovery, except in special cases.

11.11.5 Monitoring anticoagulant therapy

1. Check the following hemostasis parameters at least every 48 hours in all hospitalised patients: platelet count, PT, APTT, Fibrinogen and D-dimer.

2. In severe cases, in the event of clinical worsening, thrombocytopenia and/or reduced fibrinogen concentration, fibrin monomers, factors II and V, and antithrombin should also be monitored.

3. In the event of thrombosis in a patient under 50 with no additional risk factors, perform a thrombophilia work-up (SAPL, assay of antithrombin inhibitors, protein C, protein S, test for FV Leiden and FII G20210A variant) (this test is not urgent).

11.11.6 Vitaminotherapy

1) Vitamin C

Vitamin C, or L-ascorbic acid, is an active organic substance usually present in low doses in the human body. However, like other vitamins and trace elements, vitamin C is essential for maintaining the body's vital balance.

L-ascorbic acid concentrates and accumulates in leukocytes, lymphocytes and macrophages. The chemotactic activity of these innate immune system cells (non-antigen-specific) is rapidly amplified, as is the phagocytic activity of macrophages, neutrophils and natural killer (NK) cells, with an acceleration in lymphocyte proliferation. These immunomodulatory properties in patients suffering from viral infection are also reflected in an increase in the production of interferons a and 6^e f a sub-regulation of the synthesis of pro-inflammatory cytokines.

Intravenous vitamin C helps to boost the immune response, theoretically reducing cytokine release syndrome and increasing antiviral capacity.

2) Vitamin D

Some studies have shown that people hospitalised for a severe form of COVID-19 also have low levels of vitamin D (vitamin D deficiency). However, the risk factors for developing severe COVID-19 are the same as those for developing vitamin D deficiency, so it is difficult to say whether vitamin D deficiency itself is a risk factor for severe COVID-19. Risk factors include poor general health, poor diet and pre-existing health problems such as diabetes, liver and kidney disease.

Vitamin D is important for healthy bones, teeth and muscles. It helps regulate blood sugar levels, the heart and blood vessels, as well as the lungs and respiratory tract. It also plays a role in strengthening the body's immune system. These are the areas affected by COVID-19, so giving vitamin D to people with COVID-19 could help them recover more quickly or reduce the risk of a severe form.

3) Vitamin B6

Vitamin B6 (pyridoxine) could help to prevent severe forms of COVID-19 and its complications, including cytokine storms. Vitamin B6 could also dissolve the blood clots frequently associated with death from COVID-19. While little research has yet been done into the effects of B6 in preventing COVID-19

11.11.7 Zinc

Zinc is an essential trace element. It is present in very small quantities in the body (around 2 g), with a normal plasma concentration of 11 to 20 pmol/L. This concentration is maintained by dietary intake. At this concentration, zinc is involved in processes such as cell replication, DNA protection and hormone regulation. Zinc is renowned for its anti-inflammatory, antioxidant and immune-boosting properties.

11.12 Primary EMS activities

The role of the SAMU is to respond to any distress call that could threaten a patient's vital prognosis as quickly as possible. Before the covid pandemic, the number one reason for a call was chest pain.

During and after the pandemic, the most frequent reason for a call is respiratory distress, with or without an infectious syndrome, which makes the EMS mission difficult because most patients have a chronic pathology (COPD, bronchial asthma, hypertensive cardiopathy).

1) Clinical cases

Mr C.F called the ambulance for his wife, who had hypertensive heart disease, insulin-dependent diabetes and a goitre, and was in respiratory distress with fever. Patient correctly vaccinated against covid 19 (first and second doses respected).

Examination of the patient :

- Conscious, cooperative patient
- slightly discoloured teguments and conjunctivae
- dyspnea, cough, especially at night
- tachycardia, stable blood pressure, *SPO2* < 85%.
- temperature 38.5°C
- Asthenia

The patient underwent a blood test for biology (FNS, VS, CRP, fibrinemia, D- dimers) and a chest CT scan.

The diagnosis of viral pneumonia was strongly suspected.

2) Results

Biological check-up :

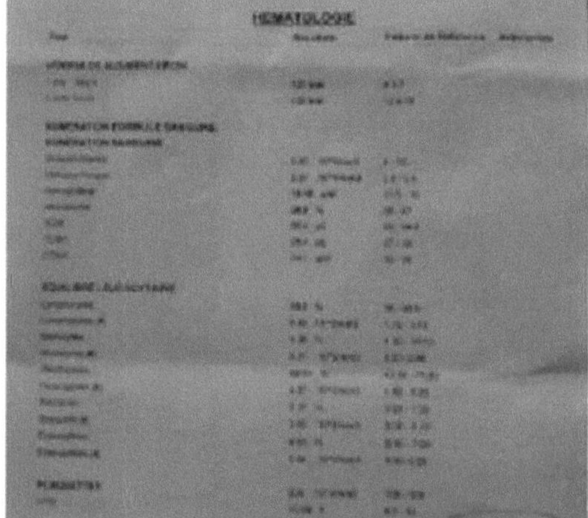

FIGURE 11.6

Severe inflammatory syndrome (highly accelerated VS, increased CRP)

Chest scan :

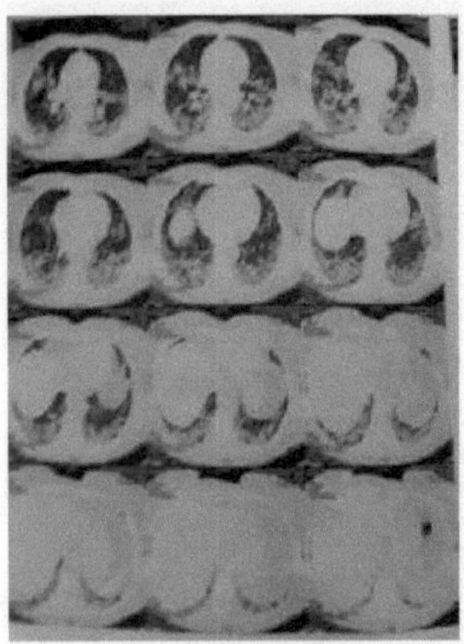

FIGURE 11.7

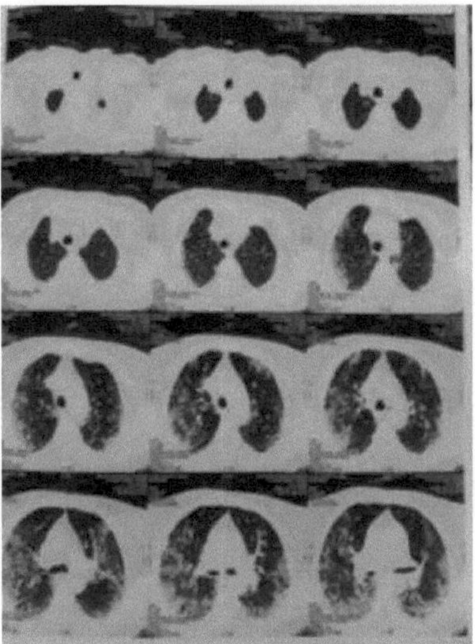

FIGURE 11.8

A ground-glass image suggestive of covid 19 pneumonia, in which pulmonary involvement is estimated at over 60%.

3) What to do

A) Aim of the treatment :

- Achieve *SPO290%* with oxygen therapy 6-8 1/min
- using corticosteroids to combat inflammatory syndrome
- preventing thromboembolic complications with heparinotherapy
- boosting the immune system with vitamin therapy
- reduce viral load

B) Patient's situation in her family environment :

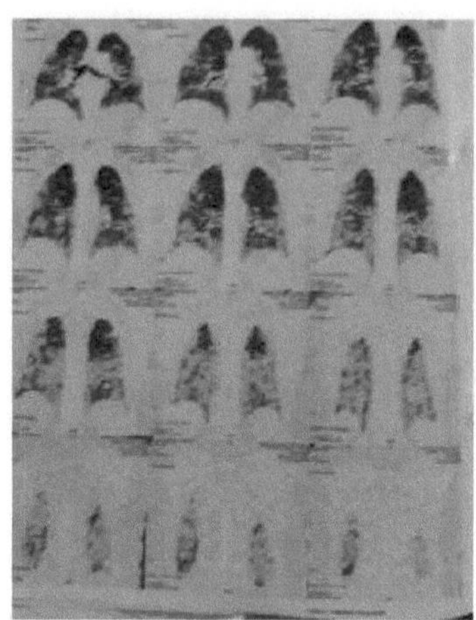

FIGURE 11.9

FIGURE 11.9

C) Data analysis :

• the patient B.N.D, aged 64, blood group A+, with a history of hypertension and DID, and a goitre, correctly vaccinated (2 doses against covid 19), was taken into pre-hospital care by the SAMU 13 and then admitted to a covid 19 department for respiratory distress. Biological work-up and chest CT scan confirmed lung damage (ground-glass image) estimated at 60%.

• His older brother, aged 66, blood group A+, with a history of hypertension, DID and obesity, presented with respiratory distress. PCR positive for Sars cov2, an inflammatory syndrome and a chest CT scan confirmed lung damage (depoliated glass image) estimated at 25%, revolution was rapid and led to the patient's death.

• The other two sisters, aged 71 and 73, with a history of hypertensive heart disease, DID and obesity, each had a goitre. In addition to insulin and levothyrox, treatment for cardiac disease included apegic 100 mg (platelet antiaggregant dose).

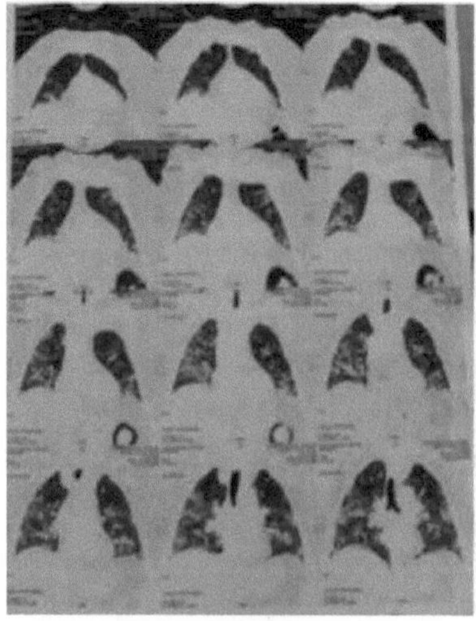

- the patient's husband, blood group B+, vaccinated against covid 19, presented with a mild form of covid 19 treated as an outpatient with a favourable outcome and no complications.
- The husband's older brother, with blood group 0+ and vaccinated against covid 19 (Neo colic), showed no signs of covid 19.
- The patient's daughter, aged 39, blood group A+, unvaccinated and with a history of thyroid disease, presented with a mild form of covid 19 and was treated as an outpatient.

D) Conclusion:

People with blood group A+ in this family are most at risk of developing severe or critical forms of covid 19.

Group 0+ members of this family are less exposed to severe forms of the disease. The person with blood group O+, despite his colonic pathology, but vaccinated, did not present any form of covid 19.

The beneficial effect of aspegic in anti-platelet doses prevents the disease progressing to the severe form.

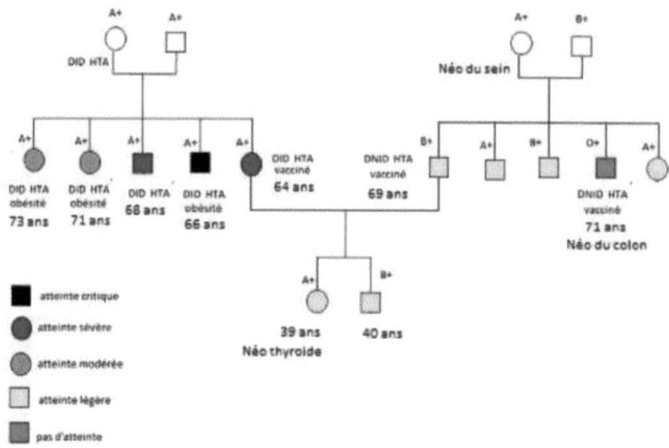

FIGURE 11.11

The benefits of vaccination in reducing the risk of hospitalisation in intensive care.

E) Treatment received by the patient :
- half-seated position
- Oxygen therapy: nasal tube 8 1/min until *SPO2* 90 is achieved
- antibiotic therapy :
— ciprolan 500 mg, 1 tablet twice a day
— zithromax tablet 250 mg :
2 tablets a jl
1 jl tablet at d5
- corticotherapie : dexamethazone injectable 6mg IV daily
- anticoagulant: lovenox 0.6 mg subcutaneous
- vitamin therapy and rehydration

This treatment was started pre-hospital and continued after hospitalisation on a covid 19 ward.

F) Evolution :

A favourable evolution towards Γ improvement of the clinical and biological signs after one week of hospitalisation, with the exception of a hyperglycemia probably linked to the corticotherapie and corrected by adapted doses of rapid-acting insulin.

11.13 Secondary EMS activities

The secondary activity of the SAMU is to provide intra-hospital transfers of patients from one department to another or from one department to a radiolgy exploration unit.

During the covid 19 epidemic, the SAMU was mobilised to carry out this task, as shown in the figures below.

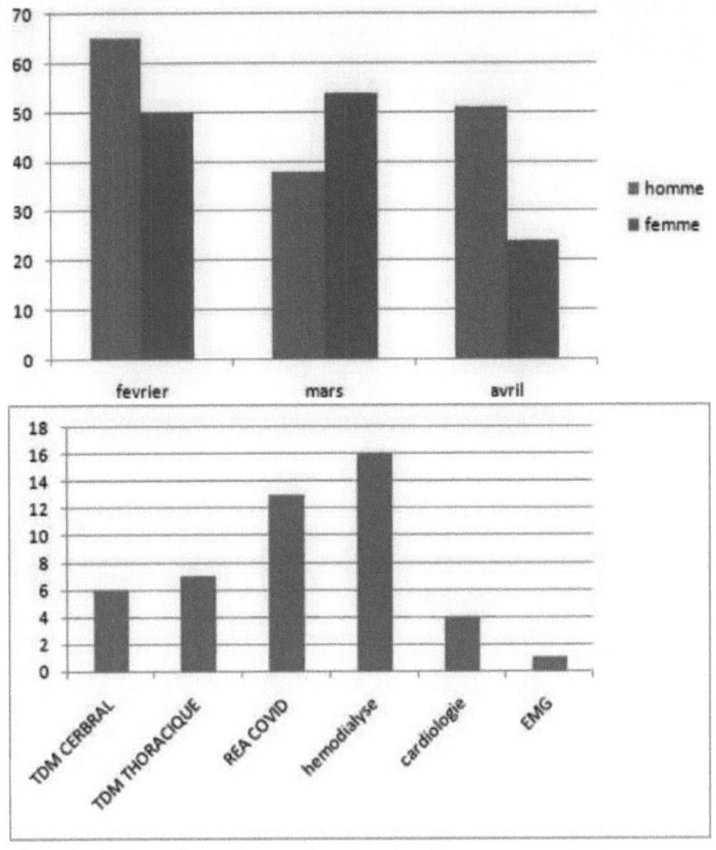

FIGURE 11.13

Figures 11.12 and 11.13 show the activity of the SAMU (inter-hospital transfer of patients hospitalised in the covid 19 service for the months of February, March and April 2021).

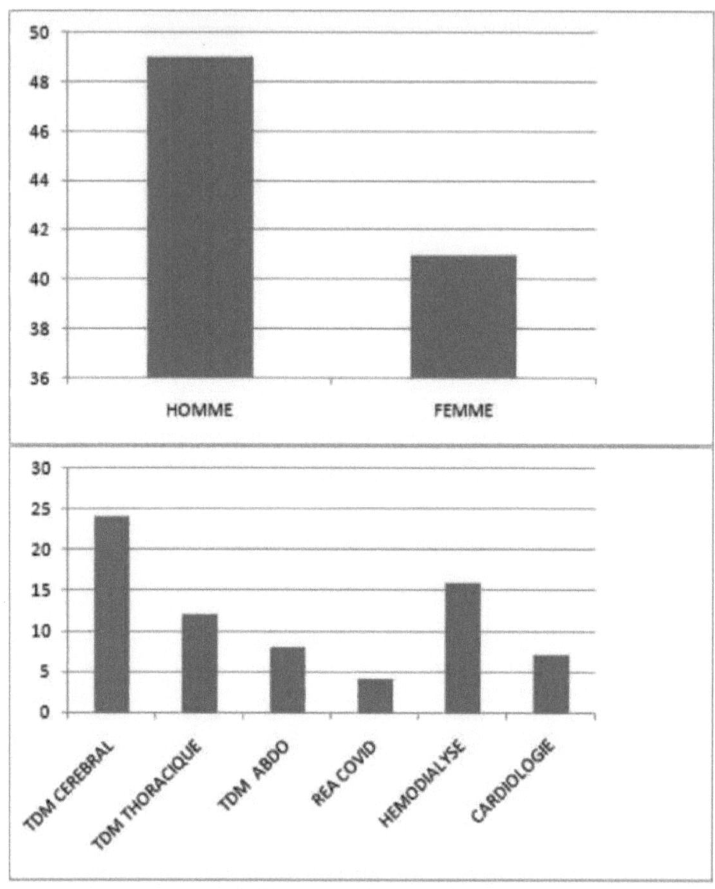

FIGURE 11.15

Figures 11.14 and 11.15 show the same activity for January 2022.

Bibliography

http://campus.cerimes.fr/histologie-et-embryologie-medical / teaching/embryo-12 /site/ht ml /1. html

http ://e.carabin.free.fr/pcem2/roneo/eiaresp/embryo/respembryol.htm

https :I/www.msdmanuals.com/fr/accueil/troubles-pulmonaires- et-des-voies-aeriennes/biologie-des-poumons-et-des-voies- respiratoires

https ://www.assistancescolaire.com/eleve/lST2S/biologie-et-human-physiology / revise-the-course

https ://microbiologiemedicale.fr/anatomie-appareil-respiratoire/

https://www.doctissimo.fr/html/sante/atlas/fiches-corps-human/respiratory-device.htm

https ://www.universalis.fr/encyclopedie/respiratoire-appareil-anatomy/

anatomy of the respiratory systemFigure(Blausen gallery 2014)

Bensouag, RESPIRATORY PHYSIOLOGY, University of Setif

http ://campus.cerima.fr

physiopathology sofia medicaliste.fr

fmedecine-univ.dz

http ://snv.batna.dz.prof.mouffouk

https :/1www.em-consulte.com/article/10863/physiopathologie-de- 1-insuffisance-respiratoire-me

https ://www.chuv.ch/fr/chirurgie-thoracique/cht-home/patients- et-famille/affections-du-thorax/autres-affections/pneumothorax

https://www.doctissimo.fr/html/sante/encyclopedie/sa-1600-pneumothorax.htm

https ://www.passeportsante.net/fr/Maux/Problemes/pneumothorax

https ://www.lesouffle.org/2019/07/30/pneumothorax-treatments/

https :/ /www.msdmanuals.com/fr/professional/troubles-pulmonary/broncho-pneumopathy-chronic-obstructive-and-appearing-disorders/broncho-pneumopathy-chronic-obstructive- bpco

https ://www.ameli.fr/assure/sante/themes/bpco-bronchite-chronique/comprendre-bp co

https://www.has-sante.fr/jcms/p-3118949/fr/les-traitements-medicamenteux-de-la-bpco

https : / / sfar.org/asthme-aigu-grave

https ://www.revmed.ch/revue-medicale-suisse/2011/revue-medical-switzerland-322/treatment-of-1-acute-asthma-in-emergencies

https ://asthma.ooreka.fr/astuce/voir/523077/asthme-aigu-grave

https://thoracotomie.com/2012/08/04/volet-costal-ou-volet-thoracic /

https://www.chuv.ch/fr/chirurgie-thoracique/cht-home/patients-and-family/thoracic-affects/thoracic-trauma / fracture-dune-cote

https ://sofia.medicalistes.fr/spip/IMG /pdf/trauma-thoracic.pdf

https ://www.has-sante.fr/jcms/pprd-2974771/fr/cancer-broncho- lung-care-course-must-preserve-priority-quality-of-life

https://www.has-sante.fr/upload/docs/application/pdf/2013-10/guide-k-bronchopulmonary-finalweb-091013.pdf

https ://ressources-aura.fr/wp-content/uploads/2018/07/Bronchopulmonary-cancers-From-diagnosis-to-follow-up-20161129.pdf

https ://bronchitis.ooreka.fr/understand/oap-oedeme-pulmonary

Item 250 : (Acute pulmonary edema), Support de Cours, College National des Enseignants de Reanimation Medicale, Universite Medicale Virtuelle Francophone, 2010/2011

https :I/www.ameli.fr/assure/sante/urgence/pathologies/embolie- lung.

https ://www.orkyn.fr/mon-traitement-suivi-domicile-insuffisance- respiratory / diagnosis-linsufficiency-respiratory

Y.Aujard, A. Bourillon and J.Gaudelus. Pediatrie. Berti editios, 1994

H. Arzouq.Reanimation pediatrique a 1'usage de 1'urgentiste. VG edition.

https ://www.orkyn.fr/mon-traitement-suivi-domicile-insuffisance-respiratory / respiratory-diagnosis-insufficiency

https ://www.eni-consulte.eom/article/56071/insuffisance-respiratoire-aigue- diagnostic-et-trai

https ://pap-pediatrie.fr/allergo-pneumo/detresse-respiratoire-aigue-de-zlenfant

https ://en.pap-pediatrie2-poc.elsevier.cc/consulter/allergo-pneumo/detresse- respiratoire-aigue-de-lenfant

https ://sofia.medicalistes.fr/spip/IMG/pdf/detresse-respiratoire-du-new-CHU-Pellegrin-Bordeaux-.pdf

https ://www.larevuedupraticien.fr/article/detresse-respiratoire-aigue-du-infant-of-child-and-adult-part-child

https ://rea.revuesonline.com/articles/lvrea/pdf/2018/01/lvrea-2018- sprrea001250.pdf

https://www.pharmaciengiphar.com/maladies/troubles-respiratory / respiratory-insufficiency / respiratory-insufficiency-causes

https ://sofia.medicalistes.fr/spip/IMG/pdf/detresse-respiratoire-aigue-desmettre-1442330452.pdf

https ://www.sfmu.org/upload/70-formation/02-eformation/02-congress/emergencies / emergencies2013 / data / pdf/101-Lanipasona.pdf

https ://wikimedi.ca/wiki/Detresse-respiratoire-en-pediatrie-(approche-clinical)

https ://www.msdmanuals.com/fr/professional/reanimation/insuffisance-respiratory-and-mechanical-ventilation/general-review-of-ventilation art ificial

https ://ecampusontario.pressbooks.pub/trlannee/chapter/chapitre-3-la-ventilation-mechanical /

http ://www.efurgences.net/sefornier/cours/60-va.htnil

https ://en.wikipedia.org/wiki/Coronavirus

Data from SAMU 13 in Tlemcen

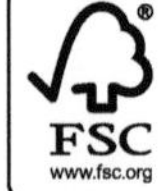

Printed by Books on Demand GmbH, Norderstedt / Germany